Answer *Yes* or *No* to These Questions:

1. I'm late over half the time.
2. I can't wait for others to stop talking before interrupting.
3. I daydream a lot and often people say to me, "Did you hear me?"
4. If I like what I'm doing, I can spend much more time on it than others can.
5. I'm at or over the limit on my credit cards.
6. I feel restless inside.
7. I have lost more than five things this week (or today!).
8. I have locked myself out of my car more than once in a year.
9. I must often reread material before it sinks in.
10. I feel very stressed out much of the time.

IF YOU ANSWERED YES TO SIX OR MORE OF THESE QUESTIONS, YOU (OR SOMEONE YOU LOVE) MAY HAVE ATTENTION DEFICIT DISORDER.

NOW READ THE BOOK THAT CAN CHANGE YOUR LIFE.

**DO YOU HAVE
ATTENTION DEFICIT DISORDER?**

DO YOU HAVE
ATTENTION DEFICIT DISORDER?

James Lawrence Thomas, Ph.D.

with Christine A. Adamec

Produced by The Philip Lief Group, Inc.

A Dell Book

Published by
Dell Publishing
a division of
Bantam Doubleday Dell Publishing Group, Inc.
1540 Broadway
New York, New York 10036

ISBN: 0-440-22260-5

Printed in the United States of America

Published simultaneously in Canada

November 1996

10   9   8   7   6   5   4   3   2   1

OPM

616.85

Dedicated to Mom,
Who has always been there for me,
And to Dad,
Who is paying attention better than ever before.

Contents

DO YOU HAVE
ATTENTION DEFICIT DISORDER?

Preface

The overall purpose of this book is to make accessible the relatively newly considered diagnosis of adult attention deficit disorder. Because this book is written for the general public, many of the concepts and research summaries have been simplified to make them more accessible. I have done my best in this regard, but some points may fall short of the most exacting scientific standards. If there are mistakes, I apologize, and in the interest of my own professional development and that of future readers, I welcome any possible corrections.

Since this book is intended for the general reader, I have avoided the traditional scientific practice of citing references in the text. However, the reference list at the back of the book cites all material discussed in the text and offers the interested and perhaps scholarly reader an overview of the major research and important books and articles in the field.

The field of attention deficit disorder, especially with respect to adults, is in tremendous flux. The future not only may change the content and texture of knowledge about the causes of ADD and its most effective treatments, but may also offer entirely new ways of thinking about the fascinating and challenging set of problems faced by so many people. We have much to look forward to.

Acknowledgments

I would like to thank some mentors who over the years have not only imparted their knowledge but have given me inspiration that one could be a psychologist with integrity. The cooperation of my colleagues has been beneficial both in writing this book and during the twenty years in which I have worked in the field of neuropsychology—with challenging patients whose brains are "different." I cannot mention all those wonderful people who have helped me, but here are a few.

I have been fortunate to have worked with some pioneers in neuropsychology over the years. All of them have been generous with their knowledge and time: Dr. Rolland Parker, in the field of Mild Head Injury; Doctors Yehuda Ben-Yishay and Leonard Diller, at NYU Medical Center; Dr. Steve Mattis, who introduced me to neuropsychology; and Dr. Ralph Reitan, who has shown me the meaning of integrity in neuropsychology.

In the area of psychotherapy I have been blessed to know and work with some giants in the field: Doctors Arnold Lazarus, Herb Fensterheim, Nick Cummings, Paul Wachtel, Jay Haley, Terry Anderson, and many others. Their generous spirits and integrity have always been truly inspiring.

In the field of ADD I have gained much from Doctors Ned Hallowell and John Ratey; Richard Carlton, M.D., who provided me with important information on Feingold's theories; and Ivan Goldberg, M.D., who gave us permission to include his assessment measure. I wish to thank the many psychopharmacologists here in New York City with whom I have worked. I also thank my brother, Dr. William Thomas, for his detailed explanation of many ideas in psychopharmacology.

And I especially thank Paul Jaffe and the Manhattan Adult ADD Support Group. His masterful direction of this group has helped more people than he will ever know, and his contributions to the field of adult ADD are praiseworthy.

Many people have assisted with research on this book, including David Sutterth, M.D., who reviewed the chapter on medications and provided advice on some medical issues. Thanks also to Lisa Poast of the Adult ADD Association in Bellingham, Washington, for providing names of organizations and leaders of adult ADD support groups nationwide.

Thanks also to Colleen Alexander, author of *ADHD and Teens: A Parent's Guide to Making It Through the Tough Years;* Joseph Kandel, M.D., of the Neurology Center in Naples, Florida; Charlotte Newhart of the American College of Obstetricians and Gynecologists in San Francisco, California; and Susan Sussman, codirector of the National Coaching Network.

I would also like to thank the library staff at the DeGroodt Library in Palm Bay, Florida, for their assistance, particularly Megan McDonald, Marie Faure, and Pam Hobson. In addition, Shirley Welch of the Central

Brevard Library and Reference Center in Cocoa, Florida, provided help with library research.

I want to acknowledge Scott William Gremmel for his help with the editing process and for his many useful suggestions. The responsibility for mistakes and omissions is mine. I also want to thank my editor, Gary M. Krebs, for his patience and excellent suggestions, and The Philip Lief Group for making this book possible.

Finally, to my many patients with ADD: You have given me a great deal. Especially to A ____ , who coined the term *Brain-os;* and to P ____ , who introduced me to this fascinating field.

All of my patients have taught me so much about ADD, and what works and doesn't work for them. Their candid information and responses to strategies developed in therapy sessions have given me an in-depth understanding of this problem, as well as many of the ideas contained in this book.

—James Lawrence Thomas, Ph.D.
—Christine A. Adamec

The names of those who in their lives fought for life,
Who wore at their hearts the fire's center,
Born of the sun they traveled a short while towards the
    sun,
And left the vivid air signed with their honor.

—STEPHEN SPENDER (1909–1995)

Introduction

Do *you* have attention deficit disorder (ADD)? You have probably chosen this book because you're wondering if you or someone close to you has attention deficit disorder. What are the symptoms of this often-discussed diagnosis? What are the behaviors? How do *you* know if you have ADD? And what do you do if you learn that you *do* have it? And is the news always bad: Is there anything *good* about ADD? Actually, there are some advantages to having ADD, according to adults with ADD as well as the professionals who treat them. So, in addition to keeping a positive expectation alive, a sense of healthy curiosity is highly recommended.

Attention deficit disorder is a very hot topic today, and some people even argue that ADD is so discussed that it is simply the latest trendy "disease du jour." Next year there will be another diagnosis on which to focus. I don't share this belief. The fact is that ADD affects millions of children; and over the past decade we have begun to recognize that large numbers of adults, often parents of children with ADD, are affected as well.

According to several experts, such as psychologist and researcher Russell Barkley, there are at least 2 million children in the United States with ADD. And, Barkley observes, from about 50 to 65 percent of these children with ADD continue to have ADD when they grow into adulthood. As a result, by his estimate there are perhaps 10 million or more adults with ADD in the United States.

The organization CH.A.D.D. (Children and Adults with Attention Deficit Disorder) is more conservative and estimates that between 2 and 5 million adults have ADD. But no one really knows exactly how many adults have ADD: no census takers ask people if they have attention deficit disorder, and psychiatrists do not do surveys from house to house. So we can only estimate the numbers, knowing that they are large and that you may be one among many other adults with the disorder.

Some adults with attention deficit disorder struggle every day at work and at home with their distractibility, inattention, and impulsivity. Many have low self-images because they think it's their fault that they're late for appointments, that they forget to pick up the kids at soccer practice, and that they seem to lose things frequently. They're often impatient and sometimes spacey. Some (but not all) seem to be in constant motion. These, and many other behaviors described in the book, cause the ADD person emotional pain, lost jobs, ruined relationships, and unfulfilled dreams.

But ADD adults don't mean to be this way! In most cases, they truly love their children, spouses, and friends, and are doing the best they can. And they often blame themselves more than anyone else does, wondering and worrying what's wrong with them and why they can't operate as effectively as other people. Why aren't others baffled by organizing their lives? Why does it seem to come so naturally to others while it is so difficult for them?

Often adult ADDers carry a heavy burden of guilt and shame that is lifted only when they learn that they have the neurobiological disorder of ADD and that many of their apparent failings in life do not result from character faults.

Who Has ADD?

The research to date indicates that ADD transcends socioeconomic differences, age differences, and differences in intelligence. You can be rich or poor. You can be seven years old or seventy years old. You can have average or below-average intelligence or be a genius. People from all walks of life struggle with attention deficit disorder.

Not Just for Children Anymore

As previously mentioned, many of the people who had ADD as children did not "grow out of it" after adolescence, as was formerly presumed. In addition, large numbers of adults diagnosed with ADD were never diagnosed or treated when they were children. In fact, according to the September–October 1990 issue of *Comprehensive Psychiatry* (among many other sources):

It is now generally accepted that one third to one half of all children with attention deficit/hyperactivity disorder (AD/HD) continue to show signs and symptoms of the disorder into adulthood with varying degrees of severity. Prevalence estimates of the disorder in children suggest that between 3 percent to 5 percent of all children may have the disorder of AD/HD. Subsequently, it follows that 1 percent to 2 percent of all adults may have this disorder (Shekim et al., 1990).

Sometimes adults with ADD knew that they had ADD when they were kids, but more often they did not. This is particularly true for women. They probably knew *something* was wrong, but they (and others) could never quite figure out what it was. And even if an adult knew that he was diagnosed with ADD as a child, he (or in much fewer cases she) may not now realize that the ADD is "still there." Why? The prevailing presumption among researchers was that children with ADD grew out of it during adolescence. It was something similar to a developmental phase that one went through. We now know that this is not true for many people who had ADD as children.

Adults with ADD first learn about their own problem when their child is diagnosed with it. Hearing about the different symptoms of ADD—inattentiveness, impulsivity, hyperactivity, lack of concentration, forgetfulness, and more—a light bulb goes on and they suddenly recognize themselves, both in the present and in the past.

Women and ADD

It is being recognized more and more that women, too, have attention deficit disorder. Increasing numbers of experts believe that girls were often underdiagnosed or misdiagnosed, primarily because they were far less likely to exhibit the hyperactivity so commonly associated with ADD. Jimmy's acting out got his teacher's attention far more than did Susie's daydreaming, which is a variation of inattentiveness. Or, if they were hyperactive, girls might have been written off as tomboys. Some boys (and men) went undiagnosed as well, especially if they had the inattentive, or "drifty," form of ADD, rather than the "full speed ahead" hyperactivity variation of the disorder.

In an article on girls with attention deficit disorder published in *Pediatrics* in November 1985, doctors Berry, Shaywitz, and others speculated that boys in elementary school were more likely to exhibit hyperactive and acting-out behavior than girls, and thus were more likely to be sent for professional help.

"These observations," wrote the authors, "also suggest that selective referral may represent an important factor in determining the sex ratio, i.e., boys with attentional problems and hyperactivity are more likely than girls to be referred for evaluation because they exhibit more disruptive behaviors that are troublesome to adults."

A major problem has been that girls with ADD go untreated and grow up to become undiagnosed and untreated women with ADD. For a person who has problems with some aspects of life, it can be maddening to be misunderstood, even in psychotherapy. (See Chapter 10 for more information about women and ADD.)

Discovering ADD for the First Time

Not everyone learns that he or she may have ADD because his or her child has been diagnosed with the disorder. Others learn about ADD when they watch a television program on the topic. "I was completely amazed at the similarities between the people on the show and me. I don't get emotional often, but I could really empathize with them," said Fred, a man who was diagnosed with "minimal brain dysfunction" (a former label for ADD) when he was a child.

"I guess I never put two and two together until the television program," he continues. "Also, I think I remember being told that it would go away as an adult." Other adults learn about ADD when they read a newspaper or magazine article and suddenly realize that this disorder might explain many of the problems they have had all their lives.

So, Do I Have It?

Now you're probably asking yourself again if you *do* have ADD. You want to know right now. Hurry up! Get to the bottom line. Cut to the chase. But hold on. ADD is not a quick-fix diagnosis, and you should not expect a rapid resolution to the problem, even if you are diagnosed. Give this book and yourself a chance. I will provide checklists and discuss attitudes and behaviors of many ADD adults so that you can decide if you *may* have ADD. This information will also help you decide if you need to get a professional evaluation.

Other Problems

So that you won't feel rushed into a quick diagnosis, it is true that at least 50 percent of the people with ADD are diagnosed with other problems. Experts call this co-morbidity. This psychological jargon doesn't mean that you die at the same time as someone else. It simply means that you have a psychological or emotional problem in addition to ADD. Often both problems need to be worked on.

For example, many people with ADD are depressed, and often it is a mild, low-grade depression. It may have resulted from the strain and stress of trying to cope with ADD. Or the depression may be related to the biochemical component of your particular form of ADD.

You could also have anxiety as a secondary problem caused by the difficulty of dealing with ADD. And even when you learn that ADD is the main problem, other difficulties caused by the ADD don't magically disappear. With work, however, the problems can improve. Disorders other than anxiety or depression may also coexist with ADD; for example, Tourette's syndrome, a tic disorder, may occur with ADD.

Another possibility is that a person could have a medical problem that may mimic the symptoms of ADD. For this reason you need a good medical examination in order to rule out medical conditions before you see a psychologist or other mental health professional.

ADD Does Not Equal Mental Illness

At this point you may be asking yourself, "If I have to see a psychologist or psychiatrist for ADD, does this mean I'm mentally ill?" The answer to this question is no. Many people with problems in living as well as diagnosed difficulties such as attention deficit disorder seek help from mental health professionals. This does not mean they are "crazy." Actually, *they are the smart ones:* They notice a problem and then do what is necessary to make their lives better.

Of course, some people do suffer from significant mental illness, such as schizophrenia, manic depression, and other crippling psychiatric problems. People with ADD are often intelligent and, according to the official definition (see Chapter 5), do not have a serious mental illness. Therefore, it's okay to see a psychologist if you think that you may have ADD; and rest assured that he or she will not lump you together with people with a severe mental illness.

In fact, sometimes your psychologist may have ADD! If the doctor has learned how to cope with the problem and lead a successful life, then that professional may be an excellent candidate to help you do as well.

Support from Fellow ADDers Can Help

Once you've found a good therapist—and in Chapter 7, I provide important guidelines on how that can be done—you may also need peer support, which is where group therapy and support groups come in. There are numerous support groups available throughout the

United States, and we'll review the pros and cons of support groups and how you can best use them.

ADD groups are even available on on-line computer services and the Internet. So if it's raining or snowing outside and you need someone to talk to from the comfort of your home, you can check out some of the on-line groups described in Appendix E.

Medication Is Important for Many Adults with ADD

It's also important to note that most people with ADD are advised to try medication as well as psychotherapy. In that way, they can treat the medical as well as the psychological aspects of the problem. Don't presume that you can treat yourself. Ritalin, a key medication used by many physicians to treat ADD in children and adults, is a controlled medication (although some argue that it should not be) and may be obtained only by prescription. In fact, most medications used to treat ADD are available only by prescription.

Some experts have speculated that untreated ADDers unconsciously attempt to treat themselves with excessive amounts of caffeine (which may calm down a person with ADD) or even with alcohol and illegal drugs. For this reason doctors worry about prescribing stimulant drugs such as Ritalin to a person with a substance abuse problem; or they may refuse to write the prescription altogether. However, experts say that even among former substance abusers, they rarely see abuse of Ritalin or other medications used to treat ADD.

I know that some readers may be quite cautious about taking medication for related symptoms. This will be discussed later in more detail. At this point try to keep an open mind. After all, if there is something that can help you and it is safe, why not give it a try?

Causes of ADD

I will talk about theories of *why* people have ADD, including theories based on genetics or biochemical dysfunction in the brain. I will also explain some theories that were accepted in the past, but that haven't been borne out by research.

The child's parents were often blamed for the problem in the past. But today most mental health professionals no longer blame parents for their children's ADD. This blaming did not do anything to ease the situation for either the child or the family. The only way you can "get it" from your parents is genetically or through a brain problem. Either way your parents had little control over what happened.

Of course, parents do influence children, especially if your parents constantly criticized you because you didn't fit the mold of what was expected at the time. This didn't *cause* your ADD, but it may well have made life much harder for you. Again, parents didn't know about the ADD, which might explain why they reacted as they did.

Advantages of ADD

Although there are many problems that can be attributed to having ADD, some adults with this condition report that there are also some advantages, such as creativity or seeing things that other people miss. A recently diagnosed man noted that the major advantage is "in my case, only needing four hours of sleep a night."

Another person with ADD observed, "We see so much more of life than others ever see. For example, I was driving down I-95 with friends on a tour of New England last fall and we were looking for a place to stop and have a picnic. I suddenly saw a deer path that went up a rocky hill. At the top was a clearing that overlooked a pond on the other side and the valley on our side. I saw how we could all get up the path. There was a place for me to pull over and not have my car in danger."

He continues: "So I stopped and they all looked shocked and asked me why I stopped. I said I found a place to eat. They looked around and said, there's nothing but rocks out there. They were shocked that I saw all of that. That is the beauty of ADD."

But there is a side of ADD that also merits some caution. Kevin Murphy, Ph.D., chief of the Adult Attention Deficit/Hyperactivity Disorder Clinic at the University of Massachusetts Medical Center, says that ADD may present a hazard for some people when it comes to driving, because they may be looking at sights along the road rather than what is in front of them.

Are there any other possible advantages of having attention deficit disorder? Bill, another man diagnosed with ADD, says that he believes people with ADD "tend to be very sensitive emotionally," which he perceives as an advantage.

Maria recently learned that she has ADD and at first was not too happy about it: "I would have brain surgery if I could get rid of it." But on thinking about possible advantages to having ADD, Maria says, "I think it makes me more interesting and fun—and very creative."

The Good News

Most adults with ADD can be treated with a combination of medication and psychotherapy, and sometimes with either medication or therapy alone. It's also important to keep in mind that many have this problem.

"Remember, you're not alone," Bob points out. "There are others who feel, act, and think like you." Before he realized this, he says, "I felt like a space alien. I didn't know why I couldn't organize, stay in college, or complete a project. Now I know." And now that he is receiving treatment, his performance on the job has improved and he feels better about himself. "The Ritalin turns down the noise in my head," he says.

How to Use This Book

Most of you will rush to the checklists and bulleted questions in the first and second chapters to see if you have ADD. That's fine, but read all of the chapters because each one offers valuable knowledge and potentially useful advice for the adult ADDer, covering everything from what kind of therapy may help you to some electronic devices that can make planning and organizing not only possible but fun.

Keep in mind that no one, including the author of

this book, can guarantee that all the advice offered here will work for you or for the person with ADD that you are concerned about. People are different, and a coping tactic that works well for your best friend or your child may not work for you. Keep trying! You'll find your own unique coping style and, I hope, some useful suggestions in this book. So keep this principle in mind: Never give up!

Behavioral Markers

I'd like to introduce an idea that will help you keep track of your progress in discovering if you have ADD. It will also be valuable as you try different methods of treatment intervention: you'll be able to "see" your progress right before your eyes. This is the notion of the *behavioral marker*.

As you read this book, you will discover that there are no easy definitions of ADD. It can mean different things to different people, because in fact its symptoms can vary a great deal from one person to the next. For this and other reasons explained in this book, I suggest that you, the potential patient and ADD person, become your own advocate with respect to your diagnosis and treatment. This does not mean that you should not listen carefully to professionals; of course you should. But you should also learn what you can about ADD and talk to others who are in the same boat.

To help you in this effort, I recommend a way of measuring—and seeing, in your own terms—how you are doing and what might be the most effective treatment or intervention. This can be done by keeping track of specific behaviors over a long period of time—as you attempt a variety of interventions. As the behaviors change, you can note what interventions are the most effective. It's as simple as that. Now, what are some other ideas that are important to keep in mind?

The behaviors that you're tracking should occur frequently enough during the week that *if these behaviors improve, then your ADD is improving.* These markers should be *quantifiable,* or able to be counted, so that there will be no disagreement about whether or not the behavior occurred. For example, "becoming hostile" is not something you can count, because it is not a behavior; it is an interpretation. But "yelling" is a behavior; and even better, "yelling at 80 decibels" is a more precise behavior. In other words, you can tell if the behavior happened or not. Another way to think about behavioral markers is to consider this question: Would filmmakers know how to film this behavior if they were in the room?

It would also be a good idea to have some markers track *different* aspects of life, such as (a) lateness; (b) paying attention; (c) interpersonal relations; (d) finishing tasks; and (e) clutter. Some examples of specific behaviors that can be tracked are the number of

- Minutes oversleeping per day or per week
- Times late to work (or to some other regular activity) per week
- Arguments with mate or spouse per week or month
- Times you drift off the subject in a certain (regular) situation

- Times you complete a certain routine or exercise (such as jogging)
- Piles of paper in your room

Keep track of these behaviors continuously so that if a change results from an intervention, you will have an indicator of progress. Behavioral markers might be either small or big things. Markers of small behaviors (such as the number of socks on the floor) might be more helpful because they don't carry a heavy emotional charge; they're not a big deal.

Make up your own behavioral markers: _____ _____. You may experience several interventions over time, and it would be valuable to account for the effect of each one. So make a chart, and plot how you do over time. We have created such a chart in Appendix A. Have fun with it as if it were a game!

Terminology

Most mental health professionals and many other people use the term *AD/HD* rather than *ADD*. In fact, attention deficit/hyperactivity disorder (AD/HD) is the current "official" term for this disorder, according to the fourth edition of the American Psychiatric Association's *Diagnostic and Statistical Manual of Mental Disorders (DSM-IV)*.

What this term suggests is that until recently hyperactivity has been considered an integral part of the diagnosis. But we now know that a person can experience only the *inattention* part of the problem and not the hyperactivity. Indeed, the label for ADD has changed numerous times over the last several decades.

I use the term *ADD* because it is commonly known and also because many adults who have ADD are *not* hyperactive—even if they were quite a handful as a child. You may be hyperactive (or restless, which is often the adult symptom) or you may not be. And you may have other problems in addition to ADD. Or it could be that the ADD symptoms alone are most problematic for you. For all these reasons I prefer the term *ADD,* since it addresses what is more troublesome to the adult—distractibility, inattention, or inconsistent attention.

A few principles or themes will be reiterated throughout this book. These are meant for the reader who may face confusion, a variety of opinions, a lack of support from important people—all of which may slow your progress in discovering whether you have ADD and how you might go about getting help.

The first principle is: *Never give up.* You may find yourself discouraged several times in your journey to discover if you have ADD and then in seeking the treatment that is best for you. Some professionals may seem totally confident, but in the end their diagnoses are not accurate. Or it may seem that there is nowhere to turn for help. Keep the faith!

The second principle is: *You must become your own advocate.* You may encounter many professionals on this path, and many treatments may be recommended. In a sense you should never believe anyone totally. Learn what you can. Talk to other people who have gone on the same journey, keeping in mind that people are different, and especially that people's brains are different.

Despite this: *Be open-minded.* Many of my patients, for example, are dead set against medication when they first see me. Don't get stuck with only one point of view. Your job is to make your life better, not to become wedded to a politically correct point of view.

With these principles in mind, let's continue to learn about ADD.

1

Do I Have ADD?

ADD has been known by several names throughout its history. It is a very interesting story, which will be told briefly in the next chapter. This book, however, focuses on concrete ways of assessing ADD and practical ideas for managing it so that you, the layperson, can recognize symptoms or patterns of behavior, follow up, and contact the right professional, and—*if* the diagnosis of ADD is reached—obtain treatment that will help you improve your life. It may take several visits to a mental health professional before you can be evaluated with some degree of confidence. You may need to see more than one expert—for example, both a psychologist and a psychiatrist. In addition, you may need some psychological testing as well as trials on different medications.

This is the beginning of the road you may have to travel to discover if you are diagnosed with attention deficit disorder. But why not be well prepared and learn the basic ideas that will make your journey more efficient and interesting? That is the reason for this book. We will introduce you to some of the professionals who play a role in this field and provide you with a questionnaire that you can fill out to get some initial sense of where you stand with regard to having ADD. Since these questionnaires can be quite helpful, we have included another—but much less official—one, which offers additional behaviors or symptoms to consider. Think about noting down those behaviors that apply to you. But first let's consider the professionals you may encounter.

Professionals Who Treat and Evaluate ADD

Psychiatrists are medical doctors who specialize in helping people with mental health problems. Their training includes medical school and usually a three-year postgraduate residency. One advantage of their training is that it enables them to understand, use, and prescribe drug treatments. With respect to ADD, this is a definite advantage, since ADD treatment often involves medication.

But psychiatrists do not do psychological testing; only psychologists are allowed to do this kind of testing. This is why, in many cases, you will need to see a psychologist who is qualified to perform testing before you see a psychiatrist. If you are diagnosed with ADD, you will probably be asked to try medication. Since only a medical doctor may prescribe medication, you will then need to see a psychiatrist or other physician experienced in treating ADD. As a result, evaluation and treatment often will be done by different mental health professionals.

You may also need to see several experts for another reason. Sadly, many mental health professionals are not knowledgeable about ADD. They may look at it as either a "made up" or an overdiagnosed problem.

Since mental health professionals are not used to working with adult ADD patients, it is likely that they may view another problem as dominant. Professionals in any field tend to observe only what they know. If they don't know or understand something, they can't see or treat it. For example, the psychologist may see your problem mainly as depression or anxiety (especially if you are a woman), not realizing that the underlying cause is your ADD. How you feel about your attention problems may cause you to be depressed or anxious or to express other symptoms. Keep in mind that although the ADD may be your primary problem, the other problem may need treatment as well.

Self-Rating Scales

To help individuals who think they may have ADD, some clinicians have devised their own self-rating scales. This chapter includes the *Jasper-Goldberg Adult ADD Screening Examination,* a screening tool that is reprinted in this book with the permission of psychiatrist Ivan Goldberg of the New York Psychopharmacologic Institute in New York.

Keep in mind that this is a self-rating screening only, *not* a diagnostic tool. Only a professional can diagnose whether your primary problem is attention deficit disorder or possibly anxiety, major depression, or a problem such as hyperthyroidism or vitamin deficiency. Such problems need professional evaluation. However, this tool can guide you in considering whether you should seek further help.

Jasper-Goldberg Adult ADD Screening Questionnaire (Version 5.0)*

The items below refer to how you have behaved and felt *during most of your adult life.* If you have usually been one way but have recently changed, your responses should reflect *how you have usually been.*

Circle one of the numbers that follow each item, using the scale below:

0 = Not at all   1 = Just a little   2 = Somewhat

3 = Moderately   4 = Quite a lot   5 = Very much

1. At home, work, or school, I find my mind wandering from tasks that are uninteresting or difficult.
0   1   2   3   4   5

2. I find it difficult to read written material unless it is very interesting or very easy.   0   1   2   3   4   5

3. Especially in groups I find it hard to stay focused on what is being said in conversations.
0   1   2   3   4   5

4. I have a quick temper, a short fuse.
0   1   2   3   4   5

5. I am irritable and get upset by minor annoyances.
0   1   2   3   4   5

---

* Copyright © 1993, 1994 by Larry Jasper and Ivan Goldberg. Reprinted with permission from the *Diagnostic and Statistical Manual of Mental Disorders, Fourth Edition.* Copyright © 1994 American Psychiatric Association.

6. I say things without thinking and later regret having said them.   0   1   2   3   4   5

7. I make quick decisions without thinking enough about their possible bad results.
     0   1   2   3   4   5

8. My relationships with people are made difficult by my tendency to talk first and think later.
     0   1   2   3   4   5

9. My moods have highs and lows.
     0   1   2   3   4   5

10. I have trouble planning in what order to do a series of tasks or activities.   0   1   2   3   4   5

11. I easily become upset.   0   1   2   3   4   5

12. I seem to be thin-skinned and many things upset me.   0   1   2   3   4   5

13. I am almost always on the go.   0   1   2   3   4   5

14. I am more comfortable when moving than when sitting still.   0   1   2   3   4   5

15. In conversations, I start to answer questions before the questions have been fully asked.
     0   1   2   3   4   5

16. I usually work on more than one project at a time, and fail to finish many of them.
     0   1   2   3   4   5

17. There is a lot of "static" or "chatter" in my head.
     0   1   2   3   4   5

18. Even when sitting quietly, I am usually moving my hands or feet.   0   1   2   3   4   5

19. In group activities it is hard for me to wait my turn.

    0   1   2   3   4   5

20. My mind gets so cluttered that it is hard for it to function.

    0   1   2   3   4   5

21. My thoughts bounce around as if my mind were a pinball machine.

    0   1   2   3   4   5

22. My brain feels as if it were a television set with all the channels going at once.

    0   1   2   3   4   5

23. I am unable to stop daydreaming.

    0   1   2   3   4   5

24. I am distressed by the disorganized way my brain works.

    0   1   2   3   4   5

TOTAL_____

Note: This is a screening examination for Adult ADD. It is not a diagnostic test. Scores over 70 are associated with a high probability of ADD.

The diagnosis of ADD can only be made on the basis of a detailed history and psychiatric examination. Symptoms resembling those of ADD may result from anxiety, depression, mania, and other disorders. These conditions must be ruled out by a psychiatrist before a diagnosis of adult ADD can be made.

If prior to taking this examination you think you have a fifty-fifty chance of having ADD, and if you score over 70 on the test, you then have a 95 percent chance of having ADD, according to Dr. Goldberg. This assumes that you have had medical and psychiatric evaluations that have ruled out other causes of attentional problems.

Another Self-Rating Test

For those of you who enjoy tests, here's a simple yes-or-no test that I have designed myself.

	YES	NO

1. I'm late much more than other people.

2. I can't wait until other people stop talking before interrupting.

3. I daydream a lot, and often people say to me, "Did you hear me?"

4. If I like what I'm doing, I can spend much more time than others on it.

5. Sometimes I feel like a fish out of water.

6. Sometimes I forget to eat meals.

7. I start many projects but finish few of them.

8. I often blurt out remarks and regret it later.

9. I hate stopping at red lights.

10. It's very hard for me to tell what others think of me.

11. I build up a lot of debt on my credit cards.

YES   NO

12. I feel nervous and restless.

13. I have lost more than five things this week.

14. I can get lost in my own city.

15. I have locked myself out of my car more than once in a year.

16. I feel like screaming when traffic is heavy.

17. I forget to pay bills, even with a second or third notice. This has affected my credit rating.

18. I feel very stressed out much of the time.

19. Coffee, cola, or chocolate seems to make me feel better. They calm me down.

20. I lose my temper easily over things others might consider trivial.

21. As a child, it was hard for me to concentrate on reading, either at school or at home. I still have some trouble paying attention to what I'm reading.

22. People I care about say that I don't understand them.

YES   NO

23. I must often reread material
    before it sinks in.

24. I have trouble starting projects.

25. I tend to make snap judgments.

If you've answered yes to twenty or more of these questions, you may have attention deficit disorder and should seek a professional evaluation.

Professional Rating System: The *DSM-IV*

Mental health professionals use the American Psychiatric Association's *Diagnostic and Statistical Manual (DSM-IV)* to help them determine the different categories of psychiatric disorders. This source notes different symptoms of ADD. If you have more than a certain number of symptoms in three categories, then you are likely to have attention deficit disorder.

Other Rating Systems

Your mental health professional may use a different self-rating scale, such as those designed by Paul H. Wender, M.D.; Edna Copeland, Ph.D.; or other experts in the field. Or the psychologist or psychiatrist may use a rating scale that he or she has devised.

There is even a computer program that mental health professionals can purchase to help with the rating and evaluation of children and adults with attention deficit disorder—Attention Please, developed by Attention Please, Inc., in Oakbrook Terrace, Illinois. It's likely that other tests and rating systems will be developed as the problem of attention deficit disorder continues to gain more recognition and diagnostic criteria are refined.

For information on how a mental health professional determines whether or not you have ADD, be sure to read Chapter 5.

2

What Is Attention Deficit Disorder?

Dr. George Still was probably the first to acknowledge what we now call ADD. He observed this problem among a group of children in London, England, back in 1902. At that time the problem was perceived as a moral or character defect. Later the symptoms that we now call ADD were believed to have been caused by some sort of brain injury, even when there was no evidence of it.

Since the early 1920s, various books and articles written by mental health professionals, physicians, educators, and others have described all sorts of causes and solutions for what we now call attention deficit disorder. (See Chapter 3 for more information about various theories on the causes of ADD.)

Despite radical swings in the theories—from an inherent moral deficiency to a nutritional defect to a genetic and biological problem, to name just a few popular explanations—most mental health professionals still believe that when it comes to attention deficit disorder, the child truly is the father or mother to the man or woman.

This points to a few factors. Almost every expert in

the field agrees that ADD usually first manifests in childhood—although in far too many cases it remains undiagnosed. Consequently the child often suffers from an overall low self-esteem and general confusion about why he or she doesn't progress in life like other children. Such a child also suffers from not learning the social skills that are so important to pick up in the developing years.

For example, when you were a child, maybe you were told over and over that you were bright enough to do *much* better in school. But you felt like you were trying your hardest. Maybe you redoubled your efforts and still received criticism and complaints. You felt caught in a bind and didn't know how to escape.

In retrospect, you can't really blame your parents or your teachers, because they probably didn't know about ADD either. But now we do know about this condition—or at least you will know about it by the time you finish reading this book—and we can move ahead from this point.

Quite often, however, the ADD adult received a great deal of negative feedback during childhood. "Why can't you pay attention?" or "Johnny, you keep losing your homework." And the ever-popular, "Sarah, if you just tried harder, you could do so well."

A key problem with all the negative feedback received by the ADD child—whether the adult remembers it or not—is that the child begins to internalize these comments, thinking, "Hey, maybe I am lazy and no good." The child may even give up altogether. If working your hardest doesn't "work," why try at all?

This pattern may continue into adulthood as you struggle to satisfy bosses, spouses, friends, and others—but the ADDer never quite gets it right. So the struggle goes on. The person with ADD tries to keep a schedule, satisfy people's demands, and finish what is asked.

But the bosses, spouse, and friends don't understand why you're late, why you forgot that important appointment, or why you are so distracted from "important" tasks. So they blame you. This situation can be changed if you learn to understand your ADD and to deal with it. And you can tell others about it so that they can understand. Self-understanding can be a great help in relieving inner stress.

In some cases, the adult with ADD really does not remember past problems with school, family, and friends. For this reason, it may be a good idea to talk to the adult's family members. If the mental health professional interviews family members of an adult coming for help with ADD, the process can clarify the person's history. I have had many patients interview their parents, and sometimes their brothers and sisters, in order to gain some understanding of what they were like as children.

This process can be very illuminating. What is important here is to try to obtain something close to an "objective" history. Sometimes stories emerge that have long been forgotten and that paint a vivid picture of what a person was like as a child. But the overall purpose is to try to determine if the child in question (now an adult) had a history that is consistent with ADD, since the history is the *big key* in determining whether a person really has ADD.

I prefer to guide the patient in a fairly structured way in this assignment of interviewing family members. During our session, we discuss a series of questions that patients will later ask their parents. Because this kind of interview is done in the service of their children's well-being and happiness, I have found that most parents are remarkably thoughtful and do their best to provide an accurate picture. Of course, I would be more cautious with patients who have difficult family relationships.

Obtaining a Diagnosis

As I have mentioned, adults often first learn they have ADD when their child is diagnosed with it. The parent notices the symptoms, behavior, self-esteem problems, and so forth. The adult may even decide to self-test with the same rating scale that helps determine if his or her child has ADD. "Wait a minute! I have these problems too!" I have heard this phrase numerous times in my office.

Often this "aha" experience leads the parent to begin the process of becoming diagnosed, which may also help to turn his or her life around. Of course medication and/or therapy cannot magically make the ADD go away, despite the hopes or expectations of many newly diagnosed adults with attention deficit disorder. It's important to remember that an improvement in the adult's life is also good for the child with attention deficit disorder. No matter how scattered and confused the child is, if the parent's behavior and outlook improves, that will help the child.

Other adults may read a magazine article, see a book, or watch a television program about ADD and the light bulb will go on: "Hey! They're describing me!" And hopefully, they, too, will seek assistance.

Unfortunately, many people still don't know about ADD or, if they do, think it's just an excuse to avoid responsibility. So they blame others who have ADD or they blame themselves if they are undiagnosed. This is a recipe for unhappiness and even disaster.

The good news is that when ADD is recognized and treated, many of the destructive problems that tend to accompany ADD can be eliminated or significantly reduced. For example, mental health professionals report that adult ADDers who were substance abusers often give up drugs or alcohol when they are treated with medication and therapy. The medication, when it works, provides them with the biochemical control they need, and the therapy provides the insight and coping techniques that are so important in managing their own behavior.

Variations of ADD

In dealing with many ADD patients over the last decade, I have been struck by the many variations of this disorder. For some people it may take the form of memory lapses. For others it might be distractibility. They may have enormous problems organizing their domestic affairs, yet be competent (at least in the eyes of others) in their work. Or they may be good at home, yet disorganized or problematic at work. Their thinking may be confused and their thoughts mixed up. Difficulty in planning ahead and procrastination are also common problems. And some ADD people have a need to seek out highly stimulating activities—even to the point of danger. Any given person may experience various forms of these problems, and in differing degrees, and no two ADD people are completely alike. This variation of symptoms—especially with respect to the nonhyperactive, or *inattentive,* type of ADD—has been the source of much controversy in the field.

Hyperactive or Not?

Clinicians today include people who are *not* hyperactive among those who have ADD when these people show enough of the other, nonhyperactive symptoms of the disorder. There are several possible variations of the inattentive kind of ADD. It has sometimes been characterized as *inconsistent* attention. One way it could be manifested is by "tuning out" at certain times. It could be seen in someone who loses track of things or events—forgetting appointments completely or believing that some event never happened.

ADD adults may not be jiggling their legs as they sit, or squirming in their chair, as you might expect with a hyperactive adult or child—but they may be immersed in a daydream and inattentive to their surroundings; they may be "zoned out." Or, instead of concentrating on what he would like to do right now, the person with the inattentive type of attention deficit disorder may be thinking twenty tasks ahead of himself. Or maybe he's completely overloaded with stimuli and is temporarily paralyzed and unable to act. You could call this a "cognitive logjam."

For example, an adult may become overwhelmed by a complex task or even something as "ordinary" as cleaning the entire house. She can't quite figure out where to start. Or when she does start, she stops after a few steps are performed—giving up because it seems too hard or because she is so distracted by other stimuli in the house. Or a person may experience "blinks," as one ADD man with this problem has described it. He is Jim Reisinger, a highly educated man who explained his "blinks" in an article in one of the adult ADD newsletters, *ADDendum:* Blinks are momentary lapses of consciousness in which information is completely lost—something like a "hole" in consciousness. (We will review a variety of lapses of consciousness in Chapter 4.)

No one knows what percentage of all adults with ADD are primarily the inattentive, nonhyperactive type. Almost all the studies on ADD were done with children who were hyperactive. But most professionals who are familiar with adult ADD now acknowledge that the inattentive form of ADD does exist and is a problem for many people.

Distractibility

Distractibility is a common and sometimes serious problem for the ADD adult. For example, let's say that you go into the kitchen to make a sandwich. The phone rings, so you answer, leaving the bread, salami, and mayonnaise out on the counter. The person on the phone reminds you of a letter you need to write, so you end the call, go to your home office, and turn on the computer. You've forgotten about making your sandwich. Maybe the dog eats the salami you left out.

As you turn on your computer and get ready to compose your letter, you suddenly notice it's raining outside and wonder if you should fix those rain gutters. You go outside to take a look at them. You notice that your garden seems neglected, so you decide to take a closer look. In the meantime you've forgotten lunch, the letter you meant to type, and the rain gutters. And you'll probably forget your garden, too, once something else distracts you.

This scenario can also be played out in many job situations, although some ADDers have found occupations that are more accommodating—such as jobs that require constant changes. Sometimes ADDers do well in sales, although they may become stymied by the paperwork. In general, the untreated ADDer is likely to be unhappy as an accountant or in a job that requires repetitive work with a lot of details.

Distractibility and inattentiveness are hallmark features of ADD, whether you are hyperactive or not. It's very tough for you to stay on top of your task, and some days you may find yourself spinning your wheels. A whole day or even a week might pass, but are you any closer to your goals? This book will help you identify whether ADD is the problem and will offer some solutions to resolve it.

Inattentiveness: Impotence of the Mind

You need to do this work, you should do this work, you tell yourself that you *want* to do this work—but you just can't pay attention. You are not hyperactive; your problem is that you are very inattentive.

Dr. Thomas Brown, a psychologist with many years of experience treating adult ADD, says that one of his patients has likened this problem of inattentiveness to a kind of "impotence of the mind." For example, if you as a person with ADD are really interested in a particular task, then you can "perform"; but if you are bored by the task, no matter how much you tell yourself you want or need to do it, your mind can't in essence get "up" for it. It's not your fault: This is a symptom of ADD.

Disorganization

Disorganization is another frequent problem with ADD. Take a look at your home and at your office. Do you see boxes or piles everywhere? Can you get your car into the garage, or is it so full of who-knows-what that the stuff is nearly overflowing into the driveway?

If you're given a project at work, do you know how to break it down into its elements, working on one of them at a time? Or do you try to do everything at once, then give up in frustration and confusion when you can't? Maybe you become overwhelmed by the different components of a project, then decide to swing into high gear—but too late?

Disorganization also wastes a lot of your time. Do you lose important items—and then find them later—probably when you're looking for something else? You probably don't have a special place for the items that you need at home or at work. As a result, that important document, or even the vacuum cleaner, could be just about anywhere.

You may have spent hours looking for your glasses, your car keys, or a book that you want to read. It doesn't have to be that way if your ADD is recognized and treated.

Forgetfulness

"I can describe my main problem in one word—forgetting!" says Andrea. "It's the toughest problem I face daily, even four years after being diagnosed. Just getting through the day is hard—remembering I left something on the stove, remembering to pick up my children at the bus stop, and remembering to get off the Internet!"

People who don't have attention deficit disorder often cannot believe that a person could forget so much, and so quickly. "I just *told* you that!" they will complain, and the person with ADD has no choice but to believe them. It seems that the part of their brain that is supposed to remember just doesn't work very well for some ADD adults. So they forget. This is why the person with ADD needs to make lists, write things down, and use other aids. We review many useful tips and strategies in Chapter 8.

Dr. Thomas Brown, at a recent (1995) CH.A.D.D. conference, called this a "file management" problem. It is similar to the situation in which you know you have a file in your computer or file cabinet, but you forgot what you named it. "You know it's in there, and you simply cannot get it out," Dr. Brown reported.

Confused or Jumbled Thinking

"I had racing thoughts, lots of them," says Sam, a young man with ADD who is a college student. "I couldn't stay focused in class for more than thirty seconds before I would drift off into another world."

Others report that their thoughts seem like a television set with all the stations turned on at once. When it works, medication helps you tune out the unwanted stations and tune in what you really want to pay attention to.

Hyperfocusing

Another feature of ADD that seems contradictory to many people is the ability of some people with attention deficit disorder to hyperfocus. What this means is that some people with ADD can concentrate very well on activities that interest them; for example, they can play computer games for hours or read an exciting new novel straight through. In these instances they may actually have greater levels of concentration than the person who does not have ADD.

Of course, hyperfocusing can have its drawbacks. The ADDer may be concentrating so intensely on a task that the individual forgets to pick up Johnny at school, or doesn't hear the phone ringing in the background—and it's the boss with an urgent request. The hyperfocusing ADDer may lose track of time while intensively focusing on some tasks.

Rushing to Judgment

Another problem for many adults with attention deficit disorder is a tendency to rush to judge an issue or situation, a tendency to overgeneralize or jump to conclusions. Rather than carefully weighing the evidence, the choice or judgment will involve simply what seems to be readily apparent. This can be viewed as the adult counterpart of the impulsive, hyperactive child.

When the adult with ADD does not take the time to consider the available information and rushes into action, he or she can end up making a wrong or inappropriate decision. In addition, the adult may become so easily distracted by the broad context that the key elements needed to solve the problem effectively are missed.

Then, rather than prioritizing possible steps to solve the problem, the person will try to find one or two quick answers to get the problem solved. But many problems or situations need more careful analysis, and if this is not done, the problems will crop up again later.

This could be true of a problem that you have at work or a problem that you have at home with your family or friends. What the adult with ADD needs to develop is a capacity to consider all the important elements of a problem, and then analyze a way to a solution. A good therapist can help with this tendency, as can an ADD "coach." (For more information on coaches for people with ADD, see Chapter 8.)

Procrastination

Everyone puts projects off sometimes, but for the person with ADD, this may be a way of life. Give this person eight weeks to do a project, and you can expect him to start thinking about it a few days before it is due—or maybe the day it is due. Then there's no way it can be completed properly.

In some cases, the person may seem to need the high

pressure and stimulation of an imminent deadline to get her started on a project—which may tie in with another ADD symptom, the need for highly stimulating situations.

But this can be a very ineffective way to live. Think of college students pulling "all-nighters" to cram for exams. And think about a person who lives this way when she's forty or he's forty-five. This kind of life is tough on the mind and the body and needs to be changed. It would benefit this kind of ADD person to develop skills to manage his or her life, and perhaps to take medication to deal with attention problems.

Need for High Stimulation

Many people with ADD need to have something going on all the time. It may be high-risk behavior such as sky diving or race car driving or it could be parties and high living. Dr. Edward Hallowell, coauthor of *Driven to Distraction*, says the person could even be immersed in a book as his version of high stimulation. The bottom line is that he is actively engaged in an activity he finds stimulating.

Difficulty Planning Ahead

One hallmark symptom for many adults with ADD is great difficulty in both setting goals and carrying out the steps to achieve those goals, primarily because of their problem with thinking only in the present. In fact, psychologist Russell Barkley believes this kind of temporal impairment (or inability to manage time) is really the key to the whole problem of disorganization, impulsivity, and the range of other symptoms the ADDer experiences.

Think about it: If you live only for this minute, or maybe for today, wouldn't your actions be far different than if you were planning for today but also for future events? Of course, they would.

This is beyond mere procrastination because, in this case, the person may truly hope to achieve something but forgets about making a plan and thus never takes one—or any—of the many steps that may need to go into a project. It's not that the person sets goals and then delays achieving them. The goals aren't set at all. Or they are sort of blurred images in the back of the mind.

The ADDer *can* think about the future, but may struggle to think about next month or next week. Or tomorrow. Yet she or he still wants to accomplish things—get a job, graduate from college, learn a skill, or do something else.

One tendency of many ADDers is that they panic and try to cram everything into an extremely short period and as a result either fail or don't do a good job. For example maybe there's an important job at work that must be presented to the big boss. He has given you three months to prepare, and what has been done a week before deadline? If you have ADD, probably nothing.

But there are exceptions. I recently saw a twenty-one-year-old college student in therapy for ADD and LD (learning disability). She was so terrified of her procrastination "problem" that she planned her projects, papers, and test preparation very carefully over a period of weeks, although not without experiencing a lot of stress.

It's not laziness and it's not stupidity. It's a problem with orientation toward the future—an inability to think about how what you do today will affect some future goal. But the general public, as well as the family and friends of the ADDer, will often look askance at this behavior and wonder how such a *smart* person, such a *nice* person, could possibly behave in such a self-defeating manner.

The point is that the people with ADD can't help themselves—unless the adult with ADD acknowledges the problem and learns and adopts effective methods of coping with it.

Checklist of Behavioral Indicators of ADD

Below are listed some possible indicators of attention deficit disorder. However, keep in mind that most adults exhibit traits of procrastination, forgetfulness, self-blame, and so forth. What is important is to determine if this is a pattern that has occurred for years, not simply weeks or months. It's also important to ask yourself if these behaviors have made your life difficult.

- You lose something an average of once a day. You find it very frustrating. One reason you lose everything is because you don't throw anything away and have piles everywhere. Which pile is it in?
- You interrupt people who are talking. You even interrupt your own sentences, switching in mid-sentence to another topic because a new thought has pushed out the old one. I noticed this rather

curious tendency of ADD adults after working with them for about five years. During the first therapy session, for example, I let someone tell me his story, and I keep track of how many times he interrupts himself. Left on their own, ADD adults actually interrupt themselves! Only sometimes do I point it out because I don't want patients to feel criticized (since they usually have had enough criticism to last a lifetime). Eventually, however, I will let them know about their tendency to interrupt even themselves, because this behavior could irritate others.

- You're consistently late. Or you're consistently early because you're afraid you'll be late.

- You blame others very frequently. It's your wife's fault that the project didn't get done. She kept nagging you about problems with the children. Or it's the fault of your supervisor. Or society. Blame is a way that people can protect themselves psychologically. Maybe it's not your fault. But it may not be their fault either.

- Or, conversely, *everything* is your fault! If you were only smarter, faster, more creative, then your life would be better. You blame yourself for many things that could reasonably be attributed to others or to the vagaries of life itself.

- You see a new car or new appliance, and you want it. Do you need it? Can you afford it? Who cares! You want it and you want it now. So you buy it.

- You wish you were more even-tempered. You may experience emotional highs and lows, somewhat like a roller-coaster ride. Your boss yells at you, and you feel emotionally crushed. Then someone compliments you, and you're euphoric. These mood swings are not as pronounced as in a bipolar disorder, but they are still tough to deal with on a daily basis.

- People become annoyed with you and you really don't understand why. You feel like your interpersonal relationships are not successful. You may retreat into semireclusiveness because you just can't figure out what people want or need from you.

- You feel bored a lot. You need stimulation and excitement, and if family, friends, and colleagues can't/don't provide it, you seek out others who can.

- You delay performing tasks that you know you have to do. As we have seen, this tendency to procrastinate can be typical of ADD. Did you forget to do your income taxes, pay your bills, make an appointment for that conference with your son's teacher? Everyone delays taking action on things. But has procrastination become a way of life for you?

- You feel like an underachiever. You "could have been a _____!" What happened? Of course, many people who don't have ADD experience these feelings, so thinking you are an underachiever is not enough to qualify you as an ADDer.

- Do you start many projects and finish only a few? Or none? This is a common problem among adults with ADD. They are highly motivated at the beginning of a project and lose interest halfway through.

- Given several months or more to handle a job, do you start thinking about it the day before the

deadline, or do you fail to leave adequate time to
do a good job?
- Do you have goals that you hope to achieve in the
next year? Have you taken any steps to achieve
them?
- Does "right now" seem so intensely important
that you don't really worry about tomorrow?

The Social Side

For an ADD child, sometimes a good day is the one
when you are simply ignored. This can be tragic: How
do you build self-esteem when there has been little social reinforcement all your life? It follows that a characteristic of ADD adults is their poor social skills. They
tend not to have as many friends as others, and they
tend not to marry. Yet, dealing with social problems is
one of the most neglected dimensions of working with
ADD people. This is why I recommend, whenever possible, group therapy for the ADD adult. Rarely are
ADD people in a forum where subtle social gaffes can
be pointed out in a supportive but firm way and where
they can pinpoint what they do and don't do that com-
promises their interpersonal life.

There is a problem, however, with traditional group
therapy. If it is psychoanalytically based, the theory
suggests that current problems originated in psychological issues of the early years—either childhood trauma
or a childhood environment that produces ongoing psychological problems. While this is true to some extent
for ADD people, it is only half the story. What *isn't*
taken into account is that the child's brain was not processing information correctly. As a result, the young

person with ADD was not learning social cues as readily as other children. So they *were* and often *are* perpetually "out of it." They are the kind of people who "don't get it."

This is not always true. I have seen some ADD and LD (learning disabled) people who are masterful in the social sphere. Or they can be masterful sometimes and absolute klutzes at other times—out of sync with the social dynamics of their situation. Also, girls who have ADD or the nonhyperactive types of ADD (the inattentive type, as discussed in Chapter 5) tend to have stronger social skills than the active and rambunctious types.

According to Barkley (1990), over 50 percent of ADD children have problems with peer relationships. This percentage may be even higher in adults. In fact, this is perceived by many researchers and clinicians in the field as the single most important area in which the ADD adult needs to work. According to Kevin Murphy (1995), some of the common social problems in adults with ADD are the following:

- In childhood the ADD person is described as more disruptive, aggressive, impatient, self-centered, and verbally offensive than others. Such children would tend not to have several friends or buddies and therefore would not have the social skills of others their age. Even if they eventually learned the skills, they would always be behind their own age group.
- Some ADD adults complain of getting bored and having brief dating relationships. They may impulsively say the wrong things, forget important events, show up chronically late to appointments,

or overcommit themselves to projects. Not everyone would have the patience to stay in relationships with people who show these behaviors.

- Poor emotional regulation and moodiness contribute to interpersonal problems. Overblown reactions, explosions of anger, failing to listen, or merely *appearing* to listen may alienate a partner or friend.

- ADD adults may lack social awareness and fail to perceive social cues that communicate obvious messages to other people. "For some reason, I just seem to turn people off," an ADD person might say.

- The workplace may be difficult since poor organizational skills are particularly detrimental. Some ADD people have also come to associate social interaction with embarrassment and disappointment, and may avoid necessary interactions with others. Poor eye contact, difficulty staying on the topic, "spaciness," and misperceiving social cues are problems that may plague the ADD adult. Not being able to have a conversation at lunch or at the water cooler may, in subtle ways, jeopardize business relationships.

Dr. Murphy breaks down these social problems into the following categories:

- Limited self-awareness
- Poor communication skills
- Poor emotional regulation
- Intrusive behaviors

Changing these behaviors is no easy task. Imagine people growing up with these problems and never relating well to their peers. They might feel alienated, isolated, lonely, or unlovable. No wonder they have problems with the social side of life!

But not all ADD people have significant social problems. In fact, some may have a unique charm that might not be appreciated by everyone but makes them interesting to be around. But even if the ADD person has social skills, he or she may still wish to improve in this area.

Other Symptoms of ADD

Dr. Thomas Brown has noted other symptoms in many adults with ADD. For example, reading and also absorbing written material may be a real problem for people with attention deficit disorder. Brown says that many people with ADD must read material over and over before it finally sinks in. "It's not that they don't know how to read," he says. "In fact, they can sail through Stephen King . . . it's stuff that's the required reading—the *work* reading—that often is highly problematic for them."

Another serious problem for people with ADD is sustaining their efforts. "They can't keep up the effort to consistently achieve," says Brown. They may also have trouble sustaining their alertness. "Unless things are really interesting, they start to slide off into sleep." He cites the case of the grandfather, father, and son who were ridiculed in their synagogue because, within five minutes of sitting down, they'd all be asleep.

Brown has also found some problematic moods that

seem to be associated with ADD. One of these is an overall irritability: Minor things really bother the person. Another problem is a low-grade dysthymia, or minor depression. The person with ADD may be thin-skinned and overly sensitive to criticism, and find it hard to avoid overreacting to relatively minor events.

Potential Problems if ADD Is Not Treated

If an adult with ADD continues to be untreated, he or she risks maintaining a pattern of behavior that usually does not work in our society. For example, if you're late for work too many times, you'll get fired. If you make promises to your spouse or significant other and don't fulfill them, you could lose a valued relationship. Because you have always behaved in this way, you may never really understand why. If you can't see the problem, it's not there. That is why this book is so valuable: It gives voice to a vague unease, and articulates critical problem areas for many people.

Individuals with ADD may face serious problems with work and personal relationships, but they can often be resolved with therapy and medication. Without treating the underlying chemical imbalance and the behavioral problems that relate to it, ADD adults are simply not living up to their potential. Eventually they might wonder, "What happened to my life?"

Some people with ADD move from job to job and from romance to romance, unable to cope with the commitment to work or the emotional dedication a spouse or lover requires. Sometimes people with ADD literally move from home to home, seeking the stimulation of a new place and new people. Taken to an extreme, this can be an exhausting and fruitless way for an adult to live. A person may come to this realization but feel trapped in such a pattern. Without insight and treatment he or she will be like a hamster on a treadmill.

Conversely, if you *do* obtain help, you can learn how to organize yourself, set goals, and fully use the talents and abilities with which you were born. Most ADD adults are bright people. When their creativity and abilities are unleashed, they can achieve wonderful things!

How Therapy Can Help a Person with ADD

Medication is often an important part of the answer for the ADD adult. But medication alone is usually not enough because the adult also needs to deal with ingrained behavioral patterns. Ritalin, Cylert, or Wellbutrin alone won't teach you how to listen to others, how to make a schedule, or how to keep appointments. These are learnable skills, and the medication often enables you to increase your attention level enough to attain them. But don't kid yourself: There is no magic pill. You need to develop your skills.

In addition, medication won't immediately rid you of low self-esteem, anxiety and depression, or other symptoms that many ADD adults experience. A competent mental health professional can help by providing active and useful suggestions. After some work on your part, you will be able to manage your day-to-day life more effectively.

A good therapist will explain ADD to you, discuss why he or she thinks you have it, and offer practical coping solutions tailored to your needs. The therapist may also recommend that you attend group therapy, where you can meet other people who are struggling with many of the same problems. Merely talking with another ADD person can be a very liberating experience because adult ADDers often feel like they're the only ones who have these problems.

Positive Aspects of Treating ADD

Once the ADD is acknowledged and treatment begins, you should become more able to change your life. This doesn't mean that taking Ritalin and seeing a good therapist is going to make it all easy. You still have to work! But with insight, work on your part, and the control that medication can bring, dealing with your ADD has a good chance of becoming manageable.

3

What Causes ADD?

Although no one really knows for sure the exact mechanisms that cause ADD, many theories have been presented over the last few decades. Today the most widely accepted scientific theories center around biochemical imbalances in the brain. Scientists believe that the brain is the source of the primary symptoms of inattention, distractibility, impulsivity, and other key problem areas.

Researchers have found differences between the brains of people with ADD and people without ADD, and specialized studies have found differences in their blood as well as their urine. For example, a study reported in the August 1995 issue of *The Brown University Child and Adolescent Behavior Letter* found that children diagnosed with ADD excreted more normetanephrine, a metabolite of the neurotransmitter norepinephrine, than did children in the control group made up of non-ADD children.

This chapter will discuss the key theories that have been put forth to explain ADD, including theories that have fallen out of favor or have not been supported by scientific evidence to date.

It's important to realize that most studies have focused on why children have ADD. Only during the last ten years have social scientists realized that many ADD teens do not "grow out of it." Instead, experts now believe that at least half, and as many as three quarters, of the children with ADD continue to have ADD symptoms as adults. As a result, scientists are now beginning to study how ADD is qualitatively different in children and adults, and some interesting differences are starting to emerge.

For example, the hyperactive child may learn, as he or she gets older, how to control much of his hyperactivity. The constant running about of the child could be reduced to an almost imperceptible jiggling of the adult ADDer's leg. Or the daydreamy child—the ADD child without hyperactivity—can become a seemingly quiet and serious adult. But this now-grown-up person may still experience many ADD adult symptoms, especially being distracted and having a hard time completing projects. Unfortunately, it is the quiet person with ADD—whether child or adult—who is far less likely to be diagnosed.

Another theory is that the brain chemistry of the hyperactive child changes somewhat, and that the youthful motor activity decreases because the brain settles down.

Although we don't have much research on adults with ADD, it's important to understand why children have it. It is directly relevant because the adult with ADD is currently defined as having had ADD as a child. Studies of why children present with ADD symptoms can explain why the grown-up continues to have ADD symptoms and behavior.

Theories Out of Favor

Brain Damage

It was presumed in the past that ADD was caused by some trauma to the brain as a result of a head wound or serious illness.

This theory was initially based on observations following an epidemic of *encephalitis lethargica* in North America in 1917–1918. Many children suffered what was thought to be brain damage as a result of this kind of brain infection. They exhibited symptoms of hyperactivity, inattention, and acting out that we find today in the ADD child. Scientists referred to the disorder as postencephalitic behavior disorder.

This syndrome apparently led many physicians and researchers to believe that such attention deficits were the result of a brain trauma or injury. As a result, in the not-so-distant past ADD was called minimal brain dysfunction, or minimal brain damage (MBD), rather than attention deficit disorder. Scientists thus labeled children as MBD not because there was brain damage but because they "looked like" those children who did have some mild brain damage.

Encephalitis is a relatively rare condition; and the forms of encephalitis that infected people in the 1920s occur less frequently today, since many of the circumstances that caused the disease have been controlled by modern medicine. Today the symptoms of encephalitis are more likely to be seizures and serious cognitive difficulties that a doctor would not confuse with attention deficit disorder.

Despite the fact that the term *minimal brain dysfunction* has been discarded by well-informed professionals in the ADD field, you will still hear doctors (often older ones) refer to the symptomatic picture of ADD as minimal brain dysfunction, or MBD. It was called minimal because there were no hard neurological signs that the brain was actually damaged in a definite way. Curiously the recent evidence about ADD children suggests that there *is* some kind of brain difference in people with ADD, although it would not be accurate to call it damage. Thus the labels of "brain damage" or "brain dysfunction" and their theories are no longer accepted by most physicians.

The Damaged Fetus Theory

In the past, some scientists believed that damage to the fetus in utero, resulting from alcohol and/or drug abuse, could cause a child to have ADD.

This theory has not been entirely discredited. But researchers are just not sure of the causal factors when pregnant women who drink alcohol or abuse drugs bear children who subsequently have attention deficit disorder.

One complication of drawing this cause-effect conclusion is that the cocaine abuser, or person who drinks to excess, may also exhibit other problem behaviors that may affect the fetus. It's also true that during her pregnancy, the mother of the ADD child may have received inadequate or no medical treatment. In addition, after the child is born, the mother may continue with those nonadaptive behaviors and thus fail to provide a nurturing environment for the growing child. However, Dr. Joseph Biederman has recently discovered in his research at Massachusetts General Hospital that a mother who smokes during pregnancy has a higher chance of having a child with ADD.

Complicating the relationship of cause and effect is the possibility that the pregnant woman may also carry a genetic predisposition toward ADD or may actually have ADD herself. If the mother has not been diagnosed with ADD, she may be using illegal substances in an unconscious effort to self-medicate. As a result, it's difficult to determine whether the genes or the drugs—or a combination—caused the child to have ADD.

According to Charlotte Newhart, chief administrative officer of the American College of Obstetricians and Gynecologists in San Francisco, the entire issue of whether a pregnant woman's cocaine or other substance use actually causes attention deficit disorder in her child is in flux; and there is no general agreement among researchers at this time.

It had been presumed, Newhart said in a phone conversation on September 15, 1995, that a "crack baby" would be impacted negatively by the mother's drug use; that would include suffering attention deficit disorder. However, some long-term research indicates that if the child who was born addicted to crack cocaine is raised in a nourishing environment, the problems experienced as a newborn may not have a lifelong impact—at least, with respect to attention deficit disorder.

Premature birth and failure to thrive are far more likely in the case of crack-addicted infants, says Newhart. As a result, most experts are taking a "wait and see" attitude before concluding that substance abuse per se actually causes attention deficit disorder in utero.

The Overdosing-on-Sugar Theory

Another popular theory of the recent past proposed that overconsumption of sugar caused hyperactivity. Take away the junk food, and the person (nearly always a child) would get better—so the theory went. Although a small percentage of children who were tested responded to cutting back on sugar, most did not; so this theory has been generally discredited as a cause of ADD.

According to a November 22, 1995, article in *JAMA: The Journal of the American Medical Association,* a search of reports from 1982 to 1994 dealing with children and sugar consumption revealed that researchers have not found a relationship between hyperactivity and the amount of sugar consumed. Researchers did find, however, that parents strongly expected to find such a link, which may explain why the theory persists that sugar can "cause" hyperactivity in people. Sheer belief in this theory, despite the lack of scientific support, may be operating here.

The Food Allergy Theory

A related theory is the allergy theory, which speculates that people who consume foods to which they are allergic respond with ADD symptoms. This theory explains a relatively small number of cases of ADD, and has not generally been supported by research over the last decade.

The late Dr. Benjamin Feingold was the primary proponent of the theory that certain foods and additives could cause an allergic response, which would in turn result in hyperactivity. In 1973 he published his book, *Why Is Your Child Hyperactive?*, which initiated a movement primarily made up of parents who found some success with his methods.

Feingold recommended that numerous substances be removed from the hyperactive person's diet: everything with synthetic coloring and flavoring; naturally occurring salicylates, such as are found in toothpaste and perfume; fruits such as tomatoes and apples; and any form of refined cane sugar, brown sugar, beet sugar, corn syrup, molasses, and honey. This diet is understandably difficult to follow in today's world. Several studies have not supported Dr. Feingold's diet as preventing or curing attention deficit disorder.

I have had patients, however, who are very reluctant to take medication and have explored eliminating certain foods from their diet. With more than one ADD adult I have found that eliminating chocolate, refined sugar, and sometimes other foods (especially those containing salicylates) can help to improve their ADD symptoms.

In fact, many years ago I had a patient who made his living in the chocolate business. He and I suspected that he would develop peculiar "reversal" symptoms about an hour or two after he ate chocolate. Sometimes he would place files upside down in his file cabinet or misplace papers by putting them in the wrong order.

One day he was driving with the windows up and had placed several large bags of cocoa husks in the backseat of his car. He made a wrong turn into a one-way street and almost had a serious car accident. I was told by a pharmacologist that cocoa husks could release molecules found in chocolate into the air—of course in much lower concentration than in actual chocolate.

However, someone with an allergy, or brain sensitivity, to these molecules could still have a reaction similar to what a person would get by eating the substance. In fact, people are often attracted to the very substance to which they are allergic, as was this man: His entire livelihood revolved around chocolate, to which he was allergic.

Although most of the medical community today does not support Feingold's theories, the idea that allergies to certain chemicals in foods—even "natural" foods, such as apples, oranges, grapes, or cherries—can cause symptoms such as poor concentration, hyperactivity, and impulsivity (the ADD trinity) might be worth studying. The Feingold Association (see Appendix B) is still quite active, and its proponents insist that toxic chemicals in our foods can help explain the more frequent occurrence of ADD symptoms in recent times.

The Yeast Theory

Some authors have attributed a host of problems, including ADD, to an overgrowth of a particular form of yeast, *Candida albicans,* in the body. This yeast can cause vaginitis or infections of the mouth, fingernails, or skin.

Supporters believe antifungal medication can kill the yeast and that a low-sugar diet will prevent an increased growth of yeast in the body. However, this theory is not supported by scientific studies of ADD.

The Vitamin Deficiency Theory

There are those who believe that ADD may be caused by a lack of vitamins in the bodies of people who need greater-than-normal doses of vitamins because of a genetic problem. According to this theory, massive doses of vitamins can be therapeutic.

Again, scientific studies don't support this "ortho-molecular" view, and in fact large doses of vitamins can have harmful effects on the body; for example, excessive levels of vitamin C can lead to the formation of kidney stones. Don't assume you are vitamin-deficient until you consult your physician.

The Inner Ear Theory

Proponents of this theory believe that ADD is caused by an imbalance in the inner ear, which, if corrected, will alleviate the symptoms of ADD. Supporters use medications such as antimotion sickness drugs. To date, researchers have not found strong evidence to support this theory.

The Social Change Theory

There are those who speculate that our society as a whole is an ADD society, with its fast food, fax machines, ATMs, and quick fixes for many problems. People want what they want *right now.* Social scientists thus theorize that our culture as a whole induces people to become ADD in order to adapt.

The problem with this theory is that ADD is not an adaptive response. Ask any teacher of ADD students how hard the ADD child struggles to pay attention in order to attain the knowledge and skills required by the educational system today. Similarly, in interviewing an ADD adult, you will discover that his or her attention problems are the source of substantial emotional distress.

Mothers also have less time to take care of their distractible child, since so many mothers need or want to work. So it may be that the environment today is less conducive to dealing with the problems of the ADD child.

Another cultural factor contributing to the general problem is the lack of discipline. Thirty to fifty years ago the idea was well accepted that growing up involved discipline. For example, students routinely memorized great poems, followed fairly strict school dress codes—jeans and sneakers were not allowed in my high school!—and were presented with a relatively clear progression of career paths. Students today are not guided by this sense of traditional life and career patterns. Faced with many more choices and decisions to make, a person might be more easily confused, distracted, and prone to impulsive behavior.

The Dominant Theory Today: Genetics and Biochemistry

The previously described theories have not been supported by enough research evidence to be considered the primary cause of ADD in children or adults. Instead, most researchers believe that ADD is related to brain-chemistry imbalances and that, to some extent, these tendencies are inherited.

It seems clear that genetics plays a key part in ADD, and scientists have found a strong inherited component among parents and their children. This does not necessarily cancel out the biochemical theory: What probably happens is that the child inherits a brain chemistry that is similar to the parent's, which results in the ADD.

Many studies have supported the genetic transmission of ADD from parent to child, including adoption studies, twin studies, and other family studies.

Adoption Studies

Adoption studies can be performed in several different ways. Problems with an adopted person can be compared to the incidence of similar problems in his biological family. Thus, for example, if there is a high correlation between ADD in the adopted children and ADD symptoms in their biological relatives, it can be presumed that there may be some basis for ADD being inherited.

Such genetic connections have been found by researchers. In one study of adoptive parents of children who had ADD and biological parents of children with ADD (reported by Paul H. Wender, M.D., in his book *Attention Deficit Hyperactivity Disorder in Adults*), researchers found that 25 percent of the biological parents were alcoholics, as opposed to 8 percent of the adoptive parents. (It's also true that adoptive parents are carefully screened and thus are less likely to exhibit pathological tendencies.) Since alcohol abuse is one problem that adults with ADD may face, researchers other than Wender speculated that there was a genetic link between the biological parents and their children's ADD.

In another study of adoptive parents—also reported by Wender in his book—the researcher looked at three groups: the adoptive parents of children with ADD, the biological parents of children with ADD, and the biological parents of children without ADD. The researcher found an alcoholism level of 33 percent in the biological parents of ADD children, 10 percent in the control group, and 5 percent in the adoptive-parent group. This suggests a genetic connection, since the parents of children with ADD had a much higher rate of alcoholism than did the adults without genetic ties.

Did the alcoholic parents somehow cause their children to become ADD prenatally? Or were the alcoholic parents themselves people with ADD? These questions remain unanswered and require further research.

In yet another study of adopted adults, researchers looked at problems in the biological parents. They found that when the biological parents were alcoholics, the adopted children were five times more likely to be hyperactive as those whose parents were not alcoholic. This does not necessarily mean that alcoholism causes ADD. Nor does it mean that if you have ADD, you are doomed to a life of alcoholism. But it may mean that some alcoholic people have ADD and are attempting to self-medicate. It is only fair to note that other researchers have not found a strong connection between alcoholism and ADD.

It must be stressed that specialized studies involving adoption, twins who are separated, and biological and adoptive parents are too complex for extensive analysis in this book. Those who are interested may consult the recent book *Attention Deficit Hyperactivity Disorder in Adults,* by Paul Wender, one of the major researchers in the field.

Twin Studies and Family Studies

Twin studies have also indicated a genetic connection. When looking at twins, researchers have observed that if one twin has ADD, there is a high probability that the other twin will also have ADD.

Family studies look at intact families and compare the incidence of ADD in the parent and in the child. Again researchers have found a strong correlation.

What does all of this mean to you? As you learn more about ADD, you might look around at your family—or ask questions about long-lost relatives. Are the same symptoms present? Did you inherit some of the ADD traits that were present in your gene pool? Again, look at the positive side: Some of the ADD characteristics may be beneficial, such as high energy, creativity, or curiosity. And if you have inherited some negative traits, at least you don't have to blame it on your weak "character."

Environment Must Be Considered

It's also important to appreciate that ADD may be affected by the environment. Although "bad parenting" does not *cause* a child to have ADD—or to grow up into an ADD adult—a negative environment can contribute to such problems as low self-esteem. Many adults with ADD say that although they tried their best, their parents, teachers, and others often criticized them as not really trying; and many times they were labeled underachievers, even stupid or lazy. Those labels hurt, and the hurt can continue into adulthood.

The impact of the environment is important in another way: Children with ADD respond much better to a firmly structured environment than to a loosely structured one. If these children were parented by adults who did not provide a strong structure, and if they were taught in school by teachers who did not set clear boundaries, they may have been damaged psychologically. The old-fashioned discipline of doing certain tasks within set time frames, for example, probably works best for ADD children. A good environment can't "cure" ADD in the child or the adult. But it can help a great deal.

A Retrospective Look

One way for you to consider whether or not you may have had ADD as a child is to try to remember how you felt then. Were you constantly told to "try harder" and to "do better"? Did you feel you were already struggling to do your best? Were your parents frequently called by your teachers, who told them that you were performing below your potential? Did you spend a lot of time in detention for not completing your work or for acting up and being a behavior problem? Or both?

Did you find yourself wanting to do "better," but baffled as to what that meant and how it could be achieved? If you answer yes to some of these questions, your answer could lie in the ADD diagnosis.

If you look back and don't remember your childhood at all—that, too, is a phenomenon frequently reported by ADD adults.

Looking at the Brain Itself

Magnetic resonance imaging, also known as MRI, gives researchers and doctors a picture of the inside of the brain. This high level of technology can measure the magnetic fields of the brain tissue that are used to create images of the brain. These pictures can be used to compare the normal brain to other brains in which some difference is suspected. It is hoped that the analysis of these differences may ultimately lead to an understanding of their causes, which in turn may lead to more precise treatment strategies.

The prevailing theories of differences between people with attention deficit disorder and those who don't have ADD center around the brain itself. Now that scientists are learning far more about the chemistry of the brain, they increasingly suspect that differences in brain chemistry may be the key to understanding and treating ADD.

Deficiency of Brain Chemicals

Some recent studies indicate a possible deficiency of the brain neurotransmitters dopamine and norepinephrine in ADD patients. It's believed that stimulant medications bring these neurotransmitters up to speed, sort of jolting them out of their malaise to perform adequately.

Many adult ADDers find it extremely difficult to believe that a sluggish brain chemistry can actually result in the hyperactivity that may be found with ADD—but it can. Apparently the brain tries to compensate for the missing chemicals by driving the body to hyperactivity—in those who are hyperactive.

Some scientists also believe that the neurotransmitter serotonin is implicated in ADD, especially when the person is hyperactive and aggressive. More research needs to be done in this area of biochemistry to pinpoint the precise brain mechanisms.

According to an article in the August 1995 issue of *Psychiatry,* researchers have also found significant differences in the blood chemistry of ADD children compared with children without ADD, particularly in blood proteins involved in fighting infection (Warren et al., 1995). The children with ADD had low levels of the particular blood protein. In addition mothers of the children with ADD also had significantly low levels of the blood protein compared with the mothers of non-ADD children. The researchers speculated that a low level of the protein could be a genetic marker for ADD.

Dysfunction in the Frontal Lobes of the Brain

Recent studies of people with ADD have used positron emission tomography (PET), a special imaging process measuring the metabolism of the brain that is more sophisticated than the CAT scan. These studies have revealed that low levels of energy are found in some parts of the ADDer's brain compared with that of normal people.

The frontal lobes of the cerebral cortex seem to be the area most involved. It is believed that this part of the brain is important in paying attention and for cognitive abilities related to making plans. If these areas do not get enough metabolic activity, or energy, the result may be symptoms of ADD.

In 1990, Alan Zametkin discovered that less glucose

was metabolized by the brains of people with ADD compared with subjects who did not have ADD. Researchers speculated that the lower levels of glucose result in less attentiveness because the brain is not stimulated sufficiently.

Studies have also revealed that people with ADD have lower electrical and blood levels in their frontal lobes than do other adults or children who don't have ADD.

When magnetic resonance imaging (MRI) studies were performed on a sample of children with ADD, researchers discovered that certain parts of the brain (portions of the corpus callosum, which connects the two hemispheres) were smaller in the children with ADD than in the children who did not have ADD.

What behaviors might go along with these brain differences? Martha Denckla, M.D. (1991), suggests that people with ADD lack some degree of executive function, thought by most neuroscientists to be a frontal-lobe function. This might be manifested as a lack of momentum when such people are no longer stimulated by an idea or task. It is not so much their inability to organize or pay attention as it is the inability to mobilize, activate, and sustain functioning over time.

So, according to recent research in neuroscience, we have discovered that the brains of people with ADD—at least the brains that were tested—showed some differences compared with people without ADD. These differences may lead to greater understanding of the problem as well as more effective treatment.

Other Brain Differences

Some researchers have speculated that the nucleus accumbens, the brain's reward center, is not adequately stimulated in people with ADD. Others believe that the reticular activating system, a certain area in the middle of the brain, doesn't adequately perform its necessary filtering mechanism, and that this gives rise to the subsequent distractibility and disorganization of the ADD person.

As scientists continue to study the brain, and as interest in adult attention deficit disorder grows, we can hope that there will be some real breakthroughs in understanding the key interconnections of various parts of the brain in people with ADD.

Newly Found MRI Differences

At the opening session of the annual meeting of CH.A.D.D. in November 1995, Judith Rapoport, M.D., chief of the Child Psychiatry branch of the National Institute of Mental Health, announced that brain differences had been detected between boys with attention deficit disorder and boys without the disorder.

"We have found that there is a statistically significant difference in a part of the brain known to be associated with inhibition and impulsivity between children with ADD and those without," Dr. Rapoport said. Rapoport and her colleagues devoted four years to studying the children's brains, millimeter by millimeter. This study led them to discover differences in the basal ganglia and parts of the anterior frontal lobe of children with and without ADD. These areas were smaller in the children with ADD, especially on the right side.

According to an interview with Dr. Rapoport, published in the winter 1996 issue of *Attention!,* "For any cerebral function that involves some sort of response inhibition, the basal ganglia often comes into play. So does planning complex sequences of actions."

Thyroid Imbalances

Studies have found that some children with ADD are *hypo*thyroid rather than *hyper*thyroid, as one might expect. The percentage of children with thyroid abnormalities in these studies was about 5 percent, which is higher than in the general population.

As of this writing, there are no studies of the thyroid levels of adults diagnosed with ADD; however, it is reasonable for readers who suspect they have ADD to ask their doctor for a thyroid screening.

Another Kind of Theory: The Nontheory

You have seen only a glimmer of the many different theories and you may wonder, "Which one is right?" They can all be the correct theory—in different cases. What we will probably find, as the study of ADD progresses, is that some theories about its causes are the best way to understand *some* of the cases. If you think of the brain as a complex network of wires, you can imagine that the wires can be broken or weak in any number of places—but with the same effect.

Think of the wiring in a house. You turn on the lamp, but the light doesn't go on. Why? For goodness' sake, *this light isn't paying attention!* There are many possibilities. First, the light bulb may need to be replaced. Then, again, there might be a loose connection somewhere within the fixture. Or the wires leading from the light fixture to the wall are broken or frayed, or they may *never* have worked well. Or the plug in the wall is loose, and no electricity is traveling from the wires to the lamp. But it could possibly be the switch, which only works sometimes; and when it's damp, it doesn't work at all. Maybe the circuit breaker is not properly connected. Maybe the power isn't even getting into the house, and there is a break in the cable coming from the street. This is about as far as I will push this analogy. But you can see that there are many reasons why the light bulb does not work at capacity. The disconnections may occur in any number of places or steps in the process. Or, to make matters worse, at more than one place!

There is actually a scientific reason for this analogy. It is this important point: Poor attentional abilities are symptoms common to many brain problems—mild head injury, some hormonal imbalances, brain infections, some learning disabilities, some problems that occurred at birth, and, of course, ADD. This is not meant to scare you, only to point out that you may think you have ADD—and you may be correct!—but there could be any number of causes.

As research into the causes of ADD continues, it is likely that there will be a *cluster* of causes—some having to do with inheriting brain chemistry from Mom and Dad, some related to the prenatal environment, some perhaps stemming from a relatively mild head injury, some from substance abuse, and so on. Curiously enough, treatment might be the same in some or all of these different cases.

So if you ever find yourself being asked to participate in research, please cooperate as much as you can. You may be helping future generations learn how to figure out those problems that we now label as ADD. You may never see the results in your lifetime, but each contribution may help to solve another piece of the puzzle and bring the problems you have experienced under control.

It's Not Your Fault

One conclusion that I hope you will reach as you read this chapter is that however ADD is caused—whether by problems with the brain, neurotransmitters, genetic transmission, or some other cause yet to be discovered—ADD is a condition that is not your fault. You may have spent a long time, perhaps years, blaming yourself for chronic lateness, procrastination, forgetting, tuning out, and many of the other symptoms of ADD.

Of course, this does not mean that you can't change, or that your genes determine your life. It is not like that at all. You may have inherited a certain brain chemistry, but you can help that brain chemistry along by medication, by adopting new habits, and perhaps even by changing your diet. So don't give up or abandon hope.

ADD is a *reason,* not an *excuse.* Many good coping mechanisms, medications, and treatments are effective for people with ADD. If you accept that ADD is not your fault, then you can develop ways to control important aspects of your life. This is a goal that I hope you will set for yourself.

4

How Does ADD Affect Adults?

Adults with ADD may express a variety of symptoms and behaviors. Some people are hyperactive, while others are drifty and dreamy or otherwise distractible. Some cannot hold down a steady job or have held many different jobs. Others have developed sufficient coping mechanisms to be effective in their work life. The problem could be manifested in areas other than work—for example, in their emotional or love life. Some ADDers find themselves involved in a changing array of relationships as they become easily bored with their lover and are eager to savor the new.

Or ADD could affect you in a myriad of minor ways. For example, you lose your check-reordering form and then you run out of checks. So you have to ask the bank—again—to order the checks for you without the form. You can't write any checks for about a week while you wait for your new checks. But that's okay. Since you forgot to balance your checkbook, now you'll actually know how much you have in your account. And you plan to write that amount down and keep careful track. But then you forget. This is only one of many examples. A more serious financial failing of some ADDers is forgetting to pay their income taxes. This is one error that can get you into big trouble!

Life with ADD definitely affects you. Before you learn that you have ADD, life can be especially hard because you really don't know what is causing your problem, and you may attribute it to some character flaw or personal failing. Carol, who was recently diagnosed with ADD, puts it this way: "Before diagnosis, the hardest part of having ADD is not understanding why you are so different from others—why others succeed but you can't succeed without a great deal of effort, and why others are so organized and yet, as hard as you try, you just can't do what they can do."

This chapter discusses some reactions of adults when they learn that they have ADD as well as some of the most common problems that they experience.

Why are we presenting all of these personal experiences before we get to the "official" methods of diagnosing ADD? One reason is that the official diagnosis is really only a diagram, or in some ways an estimate of your condition. "Ultimately ADD is self-diagnosed," I heard a nationally known expert say at a conference, and he was saying this to an audience of very well informed people. Another reason—perhaps the most important—is that your personal experience and knowledge are crucial to understanding your ADD.

Relief with Diagnosis

A diagnosis of ADD can initially be a very freeing experience for the adult with ADD. This may be contrary to the way most people feel when they are told that they have a psychological problem. Usually they are upset. But often adults who are diagnosed with ADD are very relieved. Why? Because now, after being diagnosed, they can lay down that heavy "my fault" burden.

"I never really understood why I 'zoned out' sometimes, why I lost things and why I forgot important things like people's birthdays. Now the problem has a name and I feel so free! I know now that it's not because I am a bad person," said Karen, another recently diagnosed adult. She believes that because her problem now has an identifiable label, she can learn how to resolve it with medication and therapy.

Others are not surprised that they have ADD, because they always sensed that something was wrong but could never quite figure it out. Now they know. It is something that can be understood.

Even if you do have ADD, you can't attribute all of life's problems to this alone, nor is the entire world going to change to accommodate you. But if you can give a name to the key difficulties, and if you follow through with effective treatment, you're on the way to overcoming many of your problems.

Grief After Diagnosis

Along with relief at finally being able to give a name to the problem, adults with ADD may also experience grief. They might think about the child inside, the adolescent, and the adult who have suffered from the problem.

The ADD person may pass through the classical

grieving stages originally postulated by Elisabeth Kübler-Ross:

- Shock and denial: "That's silly! I can't have that!"
- Anger: "It's not fair that I have ADD!"
- Bargaining: "Okay, if I have it, I must be a mild case. I probably don't need medication and I can handle it myself if I read a few books about it."

Another reaction of newly diagnosed adults with ADD is to believe that if they find the perfect medication, their ADD symptoms will disappear forever.

Accommodation and acceptance of the disorder are part of the journey the newly diagnosed ADD patient must travel. Sharing your experiences with a therapist is helpful because this can foster an attitude of acceptance and balance as you try to approach your life in new ways.

Not all people experience the stages of grief in consecutive order. You may go through none or all of them, or only one or two stages. Sometimes you will find yourself returning to an earlier stage that you thought had been resolved. For example, if you find that you need to perform a task that is very difficult to do because of your ADD, and you hadn't realized it would be so hard, you could deny that your ADD is the problem and assume it must be something else.

Maybe you've gone back to school and you're having trouble taking notes. Maybe you've started a new job and are struggling to keep up with the required reports. You may not want to admit that the ADD is a problem for you, so you think that it's the new job, that you're stressed, that it's anything but your attention deficit disorder. Eventually it might occur to you that your ADD is contributing to the problem. Again, a professional can help you see where ADD is a key factor and where it is not.

Problems Faced by Some Adults with ADD

As in other disorders, ADD is expressed in varying degrees of severity, from mild to serious or disabling. In the most serious cases, adults with ADD may change jobs frequently, move often, face marital difficulties, and risk a high divorce rate. I had one ADD patient who had not kept a job longer than six months during the last fifteen years. Until he discovered his ADD, this chronic job failure totally demoralized him. And he has an IQ that could get him into Mensa!

Before comprehending the cause of the problem, ADD adults may blame themselves for their overall ineffectiveness, thus dragging their low self-esteem even lower. In general the older the adult with ADD at the time of diagnosis, the lower the self-esteem will already have sunk. This is probably because of the many years of continually assuming that "it's my fault."

Substance Abuse

Some adults may have turned to substance abuse to escape the problem that they had not identified and do not understand. This is why diagnosis and treatment are so critically important. If the adult with ADD has become a substance abuser, that problem must be treated along with the attention deficit disorder.

Previous history of substance abuse is one reason why many physicians are hesitant to prescribe a medication called Ritalin. It's a controlled drug, and it is a medication that, according to its critics, can be abused. Yet researchers who have studied this issue report that they have not seen a problem with the abuse of Ritalin (and other medications such as Dexedrine) among former substance abusers. Apparently, the medication makes the person feel well, or "normal," so there is no need for abuse. In addition, these medications apparently do not make the person with ADD feel euphoric, or "high."

Another interesting aspect of substance abuse involves "self-medication." Some ADD people report that cocaine—and probably other substances—helped them to think clearly for the first time in their lives. In addition to being illegal, cocaine can be harmful to the brain. And ADD people need all the healthy brain cells they can get.

Feeling Like a Faker

Even if you can manage the work world and maintain what looks to others like a normal life, you can still be affected by your ADD symptoms—particularly if you don't even know that you have the disorder. Some untreated ADD people can manage their careers and their lives overall because of their creativity and high intelligence, but they often feel like impostors. You might think that if significant people "knew" about your problem and how hard you must work to overcome it, they would think less of you. This is related to the feeling of not having lived up to your potential, which is discussed by doctors Hallowell and Ratey in their excellent book *Driven to Distraction*.

Work and the ADDer

The work environment can be another problem area for adults with ADD, and blame and shame can build up over time. Most jobs have certain inherent deadlines, whether they are rigidly enforced or not. They also include details and tasks that must be accomplished, whether it's filling out your time card or writing a doctoral dissertation.

In many jobs, you must work with other people, follow orders, tell others what you need to get the job done, and keep track of what you did yesterday, what you plan to do today, and what you'll do tomorrow or next week. Thus if you fall down on your end, others will become annoyed and angry with you and feel that you are preventing them from doing their job by your inaction. And if you don't or can't get your work done on time, have many projects going at once, are very distractible, and exhibit other traits of the person with ADD, even your ability to keep a job can be affected.

Researchers Gabrielle Weiss and Lily Trokenberg Hechtman have studied children with ADD into adulthood and found that often adults with ADD have had many jobs and do not attain the same socioeconomic status as their non-ADD siblings.

The adult ADDer who doesn't know his or her diagnosis and is not under treatment may feel guilty and frustrated. "I couldn't get things done and I felt like I wasn't doing a good job for the company," said Al, who was later diagnosed and treated for ADD.

The Americans with Disabilities Act (ADA) protects some adults with ADD on the job—but you have to be willing to *tell* your boss about the problem if you expect any changes to be made. Many people are extremely reticent about disclosing their ADD because, even with therapy, the shame still lingers. This may happen even if you learn that ADD is a biological problem and that it's not your fault.

The ADA requires employers to make reasonable accommodations when they know about a disability. Examples of reasonable accommodations are allowing the employee to work in a quieter environment, letting an employee come in early or work late in order to get the work done, or modifying a job site in some way. For example, according to attorney Lei Ann Marshall Cohen in her article on the ADA in the winter 1995 issue of *Attention!,* a person who receives many oral instructions may ask her or his supervisor to put instructions on tape or in writing.

Of course, not all symptoms of ADD are considered "disabling" under the ADA. For example, the disability must be one that impairs the person both on and off the job. As a result people who have mild forms of ADD may not be eligible for accommodations.

For more information contact the ADA Regional Disability and Technical Assistance Center at 800-949-4232. Another number to call is the Job Accommodation Network at 800-ADA-WORK. Two lawyers, Peter and Patricia Latham, have published a book entitled *Attention Deficit Disorder and the Law,* in which they detail how the ADD disability can be handled legally.

Types of Jobs Matter a Lot

In his book, *Attention Deficit Disorder: A Different Perception,* Thom Hartmann speculates that many entrepreneurs may be ADDers because of their flair for new ideas, willingness to face danger, and desire for independence. The very active person with ADD may have an exciting idea, press to bring it to market, and work incessantly until it succeeds. Then the company begins to mature and the ADD adult becomes confused and lost because that initial burst of high energy, creativity, and obsession (or hyperfocus) is no longer what the company needs. At this stage, what the company needs most is a stable manager—what Hartmann calls a farmer.

Experts say that your success or failure may well be related to the type of job you hold. For example, the ADDer who struggles to be a bookkeeper may face great difficulty, whereas the ADDer in a job that offers continual challenges may excel. This is because the cognitive demands of paying attention over time—as in the work of a bookkeeper—may be quite difficult for the person with ADD. On the other hand, the structure of regular work might be just what the ADDer needs in order to keep a job. As you get to know more ADD people, you will find them working at jobs that demand various combinations of cognitive skills and work structures.

Your Learning Ability

ADD can negatively affect your ability to learn, just as it may have done in childhood. According to Mary, a woman diagnosed with ADD, "the most serious problem was its effect on my learning. I was so easily frustrated and terribly impatient and couldn't bear to just sit there and go through the steps of something—not even if I wanted to. Now I still get frustrated and impatient but I have found that the Dexedrine helps." Mary's grades have gone up now, and she feels her life is much improved. (Dexedrine is one of the popular medications used to treat ADD. See Chapter 6 for further information on medications used to treat attention deficit disorder.)

Thinking and Behavior Problems

Struggling to Focus and Concentrate

"I had racing thoughts, lots of them," said Bill, a man who was diagnosed with ADD last year. "I couldn't stay focused in class for more than thirty seconds before I would drift off into another world."

Jim, a Boy Scout leader who realized that he probably had ADD after he tried to deal with two hyperactive children in his troop, said that his main problem was concentrating at work. "I would drift off during meetings and was unable to absorb information from material I had to read."

Tom was very blunt about his problem: "My brain would short-circuit. Nothing could be retained and I was very hyperactive, even as an adult."

Although no one needs to concentrate intensely at all times, concentration is an important factor in both personal and work relationships. And a lack of concentration can be annoying to the individual himself, who finds that he can't read the book that he needs to master in order to pass an important test that would lead to a promotion at work.

To evaluate your own ability to concentrate, ask yourself these questions:

- Can I sit down at a task and perform it for at least twenty to thirty minutes, or must I repeatedly get up for more tools, for a drink, or just to move about?
- When I attend a speech or public event, do I continually play with the program or move around in my seat?
- Do people in my family and at work seem to ask this question a lot: "Are you listening to me?"

Trouble Handling Details

Many adults with ADD can handle the broad, sweeping aspects of their job, but even the smartest ADDer may become flummoxed about something as seemingly simple as filling out a time card or preparing a brief weekly report. They know the basic concept of getting paid X number of dollars for X hours of work, but they either forget to do the time card altogether or they get confused by all the little boxes on the form. So they do it wrong or don't do it at all, which leads to an unhappy supervisor. Some ADD people are absolutely phobic about forms: They look at all those boxes, lines, and small print, and they simply freeze—as if they had been taken over by aliens in a horror movie.

Hyperfocusing

The opposite of the inability to focus is the ability to focus intensely—what some experts call "hyperfocusing." As noted in a previous chapter, some people with ADD can hyperfocus nonstop for hours. The classic example is the child with ADD who could play computer games for hours. Adults can hyperfocus, too, on sports, games, and sometimes career tasks. This means that they are so connected to the task at hand that they become totally absorbed in it. Hyperfocusing on an important job can enable the person to mobilize all his brain power and energy to perform the job effectively. So it has its advantages.

The downside of hyperfocusing is that the person forgets to do other tasks that need to be done. The person may also forget to eat, drink, sleep, or perform bodily functions. This could result in burnout. In more typical circumstances, the person with ADD may spend too much time on one task and forget or have trouble shifting to other tasks that need to be done.

Boredom

"The best model for the ADD brain is that of a 'sleepy' frontal cortex, a constant underarousal of the part of the brain that normally services executive functions, such as self-monitoring, emotional restraint, judgment, sequencing, planning, organization, prioritization, and task completion. It is for this reason that many ADDers seek high-stimulation situations, since it is only in times of crisis or excitement that this part of their brain 'wakes up' and allows them to feel that they have everything together," remarked psychiatrist John Ratey in an interview published in *Coaching Matters*.

Adults with ADD may also find themselves "zoning out" when a discussion becomes too technical or difficult. They may become fidgety or start to daydream about interesting times in the past or activities they'd like to try. If you've been called a space cadet or "in your own world" by others, this symptom may apply to you.

Sometimes the problem of being easily bored can extend into personal relationships. The person with ADD finds himself quickly falling in love time after time. In addition, when a couple is strongly attracted to each other right away, the person with ADD may decide, "This is It. True love. This is the person to marry." But it may all be too intense, too fast, and doomed to failure.

The initial intensity and euphoria of a new romance cannot last forever. When that wears off, the person with ADD may become bored and move on. The other person in the relationship, who may not have ADD, can be crushed. Are you familiar with these scenarios? Did you ever think that the easily bored person might have a biological, or brain, disorder?

Inconsistent Work Performance

Sometimes the ADDer can do a great job and people will say, "I didn't know you had it in you!" This is okay for now, but people come to expect you to do as well again. Often the adult with ADD does well today, okay tomorrow, and pretty lousy the next day—depending on the circumstances. Remember that many adults (and children) with ADD are not at all future oriented. The stimuli that bombard them *now*—positive or negative—often have a strong impact on their work performance; and the ADD person may become distracted or thrown off even by positive comments.

This pattern of working well sometimes and less well at other times is also an expression of the ADD person's inconsistent ability to focus. It can be frustrating because you may believe, "I have it in me to do a great job all the time!" But you can't seem to do it consistently.

Impulsivity

Another common problem of many ADDers is blurting out thoughts without censoring them. This can cause embarrassment and annoyance. "I said things that ought to be phrased more tactfully or left unsaid altogether," Tom observed.

Many people think insulting or humorous thoughts about others, but they keep these thoughts to themselves. But remaining silent can be a very difficult task for ADD adults; words may fly out of their mouths without their control.

The person who often says exactly what is on his mind may be shunned by others for such extreme bluntness, and can even be fired from his job. This behavior doesn't tend to win friends and influence people. It also causes considerable embarrassment and self-blame for some people—if they can see it as a problem! Until the ADD person can gain some degree of mastery over this kind of impulsive speaking, he or she may struggle with relationships.

But blurting out what one is thinking is not the only way that impulsivity presents itself in the ADD adult. Instead ADD people may find themselves making sudden extravagant purchases without, for example, considering that this month's mortgage payment is still due. Hey, they want that new sofa, so they buy it! They *need* it—or they think they do.

One serious problem area for the ADDer is the credit card, which provides instant gratification by allowing you to buy what you want and ignore payment.

Unfortunately payments come due, and the impulsive ADDer—lacking a future orientation—may have no plan at all for meeting those payments.

The adult ADDer may also be a daredevil and impulsively engage in dangerous sports or activities. Sometimes he or she may do this by design, choosing activities such as skydiving, race car driving, ski jumping, and the like.

Disorganization

Problems with disorganization can be expressed in many different behaviors. For example, the adult ADDer may seem to lose everything. What happened to that paper you were just working on? Did it walk out of here? No, it's probably in one of the many piles on your desk. Or you might have taken it with you when you went to get some coffee and started to talk with an associate and forgot you put it down there.

Forgetting birthdays and appointments is also a problem of disorganization. The ADDer doesn't write down on his calendar what needs to be done, assuming he'll remember it. But he doesn't. Or if he did write it down, it was jotted on a random piece of paper, which he lost. . . . Now, where *is* that paper? Disorganization is a major problem for ADDers, and will be discussed in further chapters.

Distractibility

One of the most common problems of ADD adults is being easily distracted from the task at hand. For example, you may be working on one project, but then the phone rings and your entire attention shifts to that.

The original project is forgotten. The caller asks you to perform some other task, and you agree. Then the boss walks in and tells you to do something else; so the caller (and the project you had been working on) are both forgotten as all your attention shifts to the boss.

ADDers have difficulty compartmentalizing and prioritizing their work. For example someone without ADD might think, "Okay, I'll do what the boss needs this afternoon, but in the meantime I must get this project done, and after that I'll work on the problem Mary just called me about." But for the person with ADD each event is often experienced as discrete—a single event that gets 100 percent attention from the ADDer, for the moment.

Lapses and Alterations of Consciousness

Our knowledge of the ADD consciousness is so sparse that there is no way of knowing how many people experience the phenomena sketched out here; by no means do all of the phenomena outlined below occur in most ADD people. They seem to be different variations of the broad category of inconsistent attention.

For those of you who have not had any of the following experiences, they may seem rather strange. But those who have experienced them might say, "Aha!"

Absences

One fairly common experience in a variety of neurological disorders is called an *absence*. This occurs when there is a momentary loss of consciousness, in which a person does not register any information. For example, you might see someone staring into space as if he were a zombie for just a second or two. What we professionals in the neurosciences think is happening is that a tiny discharge occurs in the brain similar to a small seizure. In most cases this is nothing to worry about. But it possibly indicates a subtle problem with the brain.

I discovered this unexpectedly after working for several months with Peter, a man who had ADD. I had completed a neuropsychological battery and discovered that he had average intelligence although he had scored poorly on some measures in the test battery. I was trying to figure out his diagnosis, and nothing was making sense. Then he brought in one of his good friends, who wanted to share some information. Mentioning an incident in which Peter had made a social mistake, his friend added, "You know, it was one of those times when you go blank and don't seem to be listening." I inquired further, and it seemed that Peter had experienced small, brief blank-out periods all his life. This helped to explain why he always seemed to be missing information whenever he tried to learn something new. It turned out to be one key to diagnosing his attention deficit disorder.

Absences do not happen with every ADD person, or even with most. But it is not an uncommon phenomenon. It could also be related to a very mild seizure disorder—which is treatable—so if you have this problem, be sure to see a neurologist, who may be able to help you.

Blinks

The mental equivalent of an eye blink, *blinks* take up a short period of time in which information does not get to the brain. They can last a few seconds (or even less), and even up to fifteen minutes, according to Jim Reisinger, who described this phenomenon in himself.

According to Reisinger, his blinks are involuntary—something like the switching of channels on a TV. He notes that this problem can compromise some cognitive processing, such as reading, and can result in failure at important tasks, underachievement, and the predictable low self-esteem. For example, a teacher is going over ten points in a lecture. The person who blinks may have taken down the first four points. When he looks up again, the teacher is at number 7. Where did 5 and 6 go? It can also happen in reading, as sentences are "blinked over" and need to be reviewed again, thus slowing down the reading speed.

A person may not even be aware that he or she is blinking, as was the case with Peter. Interestingly, he found relief when he began taking Ritalin. It is not clear to me exactly how blinks differ from absences, and many neurologists might consider them the same phenomenon.

Cognitive Dimming

This occurs when the mental energy that helps a person pay attention diminishes—something like turning down the dimmer switch that controls light in many homes. When this happens, cognitive processing seems to slow down. There is less energy available for performing a task than when a person is "fully charged." It may appear that you are not so smart or, again, not paying attention to something or to someone. It becomes harder to do things, and a person's physical behavior can slow down, along with the thought processes. One interesting effect is "rationing the output," which makes verbal communication appear telegraphic in nature.

Since this is such a new concept, and probably a hard one to test, it will have to await further study for clarification. It is interesting to note that the phenomena of blinks, cognitive dimming, and inner noise were introduced by two ADD adults who had these experiences, Jim Reisinger and Paul Jaffe. This illustrates just how important it is for clinicians to listen carefully and value what our patients tell us.

Inner Noise

Do you know what it's like to hear static on the radio, or in a car or on a cordless phone? It is scratchy and gets in the way of the talking or music. In the same way, some ADD people experience *inner noise*. Sometimes the noise is reported as "static," but it could also refer to tunes that are playing inside one's head, recurrent or intrusive thoughts, daydreaming, mental gridlock, and the "pinball effect," as if a bunch of thoughts were humming around inside. Some people report relief of symptoms when they take medication.

These are only a few examples of altered states of consciousness that may occur with adult ADD. Descriptions of these experiences are not precise, and the best we can do now is to make use of analogies such as static, noise, dimming, and the like. Research will tease out the degree to which these phenomena are similar and how often they occur within the ADD population.

Do these experiences reflect a lower level of intelligence? Emphatically *no*! I know several of the ADD people who have described these lapses of consciousness, including Jaffe and Reisinger, who are far above average in intelligence. Maybe some of you have experienced different phenomena. Keep in mind that the brain can do all kinds of things. Here are some other experiences that have been reported.

Brain Typos, or Brain-os

One of my ADD patients named an experience he has a few times each week. He calls it a *brain-o* and it is the mental equivalent of a "typo." It occurs when some unwanted behavior is substituted for a more sensible behavior. Some examples: pouring an extra glass of water into the soup mix; putting the phone-bill stub into the return envelope and filing away the remittance slip; after drinking a glass of milk, putting the washed glass in the refrigerator and throwing out the half-carton of milk; turning off the TV, going into the kitchen for a snack, and then returning to the living room without the snack.

Overloading Your Circuits

There are times when too many stimuli are bombarding the ADD person. The circuits become overloaded, and the brain just turns off. A person may be able to walk down the street or answer simple questions; but in terms of thinking something through or having an intelligent discussion—the brain doesn't seem to be working. This can also happen to people with mild head injury, except that their reactions are usually more extreme. And sometimes not only are their brains unable to think about an issue, but their bodies sometimes cannot move—as if the circuit breaker had just blown.

Procrastination

Another very common problem among ADDers is delaying work that needs to be done until deadlines have passed or it's so late that doing the work would be. pointless. The major problem may be that a person lacks a sense of timeliness and feels that she has all the time in the world to do a task.

Then the adult ADDer may forget about the task altogether, or remember it when the time for performance is past. Or remember it the night before it's due and struggle frantically to get the project done. (Here's where hyperfocusing may come in as a useful trait.)

Sexual Problems and Personal Intimacy

Even the area of sexual intimacy can be a serious problem for an adult with ADD. Experts say that ADDers tend to be either hypersexual, wanting lots and lots of sex, or they may withdraw from sex because they don't like to be touched or stroked and can't stand that intimate level of emotional connection with another person.

They may also withdraw from sex because the daily demands of the significant other become too much. It's hard enough to cope with their own lives, but to add someone else into the equation tips over the scales into total unmanageability. So it may seem easier not to have anyone in their lives and thus avoid the problem altogether. Lonely, but easier.

It may also be difficult for adults with ADD to continue a close relationship with another person, in part because they are easily bored and may rapidly wish to move on to a new relationship. They may also enjoy the heady excitement and mystery that comes with not knowing a person well and the euphoria that sometimes accompanies a new relationship. The adult ADDer may have trouble with the quiet side of a relationship with someone he knows well and may look elsewhere.

Either way, struggling with such problems of sexuality and/or maintaining a close personal relationship can wreak havoc with a person's emotional and personal life. Yet the sexual problems, along with others directly related to ADD, can be worked on and often resolved. Ignore the problem, however, and things will continue on the same disastrous course. Medication may help with such problems, but often the adult with ADD needs advice from a mental health professional to reorient thinking as well.

The ADD Adult as Parent

Another problem area for adults with ADD is parenting their children, and often adult ADDers have great difficulty with the multifaceted tasks of rearing children. Caring for a child requires not only love but also sustained attention.

If you can never play with your child or you tune out when she is halfway through trying to tell you about her day, then your child may mistakenly believe that you don't care about her. And if the child has ADD too, the parenting becomes all the more difficult for the adult with attention deficit disorder. Keep in mind that parents without ADD find parenting an ADD child to be a challenging task, so parents with ADD may find it formidable at times.

Adult ADDers have reported that after treatment they were able to sit still and look their child right in the eyes and truly listen. Think how valuable this experience can be to a child, whether the child has ADD or not.

The parent with ADD who is trying to raise a child with ADD is at a particular disadvantage, especially when neither parent nor child has been diagnosed. Children with ADD can be very challenging for any parent to rear. But, for example, the ADD parent who is short-tempered and has a brief attention span will often create, unknowingly, a lose-lose situation for both himself and his child.

Not that it's easy for the ADD adult who *knows* he's ADD to be a good parent to a child with ADD. But with knowledge comes information and coping mechanisms and far more acceptance.

Effects of Holidays and Special Occasions

Certain times of year may be especially stressful for adults with ADD. Often holidays, birthdays, and special occasions such as Christmas or New Year's can create havoc in the life of an adult with ADD and throw the person into a tailspin. Part of the reason is the extra work and details that must be managed—when "normal life" is already hard. Do you find yourself feeling very stressed out in mid to late December? Do you begin to exhibit more of your own personal ADD symptoms?

Another stressor is that the structure that enables the successful person with ADD to cope changes or may disappear altogether during the holidays. For example, family members may come for a visit, but before they do, you must get the house ready and plan for special meals and activities, all of which is difficult for many people with ADD. Holidays are also stressful for many people who may plunge into a depression because the actual holidays don't live up to their great expectations. For the ADDer, the whole experience can be overwhelming—especially because of the extra stimulation that makes it even harder to cope.

Secondary Problems for Adults with ADD

Before diagnosis, most people with ADD have convinced themselves—based on feedback from others and their own evaluation—that they are stupid or crazy or incompetent at life. They may even have become too discouraged to try.

After he was diagnosed with ADD, Tom no longer believed he was stupid. He tried out some new projects and found, with his therapist's encouragement, that he could do them quite well. He was able to return to college, graduate, and even get an advanced degree. Although he still struggled to become organized, he used various techniques to pull him through.

As discussed earlier in the chapter, the adult with ADD can have a variety of problems at work, depending on the person, type of job, boss, and other factors. No matter how hard you try to overcome these problems, if you have ADD and are not undergoing medication treatment or mental health counseling, you may not make as much progress as you could.

5

How Is ADD Diagnosed?

How do mental health professionals know if you have ADD? Even experts admit that it can be a very tricky diagnosis because so often ADD looks like something else. For example, many ADD symptoms may seem like anxiety or depression. If you are treated for such a problem and not for the underlying ADD (if that is your condition), then you will continue to experience difficulties.

John, a man newly diagnosed with ADD, remarked, "I have been told over the past few years that I had everything from a middle-ear dysfunction to major depression to manic depression. But none of the treatments for those things worked for me. Now that the ADD diagnosis has finally been made, I have new hope of overcoming it."

It is important to determine the underlying cause of a person's symptoms. Not trying to find out what causes the chronic and distressing symptoms would be similar to giving a chronic insomniac a sedative without trying to learn what is causing the insomnia in the first place. A good clinician should try to discover the cause of your problem rather than treat the symptoms alone.

In fact, this is one of the biggest problems in this new field of adult ADD. Many people who should have been diagnosed with ADD have been treated as if they had some other condition. Or they may have been told that they just haven't been "trying hard enough"— something they may have heard all their lives.

I have had many patients come to me who had been in psychoanalytically oriented therapy for years and were not getting anywhere. I found that they had either ADD or secondary problems related to having an undiagnosed learning disability. Within a relatively short period of time I set them on a more productive course that led to improvements in their lives. So it is strongly recommended that you find a therapist who is familiar with ADD and who can develop a workable program that will address the problems associated with it.

Clinicians who are experienced with ADD rely on a variety of different measures to assist in the diagnosis. You may be diagnosed first by a psychiatrist and then have it confirmed by a psychologist. Or you may be treated solely by a psychiatrist. Most mental health professionals use as their diagnostic guidebook the *Diagnostic and Statistics Manual (DSM-IV)*, published by the American Psychiatric Association. The clinician, however, must still use his or her judgment to make the diagnosis for or against ADD.

There has been heated argument over whether adults and children should have separate diagnostic categories. Experts have recently revised the *DSM-IV* to encompass people of all ages. *DSM-IV* is the bible of psychologists and psychiatrists nationwide. According to this source, the symptoms of AD/HD are as follows:

1. **Inattention:** At least 6 of the following symptoms of inattention have persisted for at least 6 months, and are maladaptive and inconsistent compared to people your age.

____(a) often fails to give close attention to details or makes careless mistakes in schoolwork, work, or other activities

____(b) often has difficulty sustaining attention in tasks or play activities

____(c) often does not seem to listen to what is being said to him/her

____(d) often does not follow through on instructions and fails to finish schoolwork, chores, or duties in the workplace (not due to oppositional behavior or failure to understand instruction)

____(e) often has difficulties organizing tasks and activities

____(f) often avoids, dislikes, or is reluctant to engage in tasks that require sustained mental effort (such as school or homework)

____(g) often loses things necessary for tasks or activities (for example, school assignments, pencils, books, tools, or toys)

____(h) is often easily distracted by extraneous stimuli

____(i) is often forgetful in daily activities

2. **Hyperactivity-Impulsivity:** At least 6 of the following symptoms of hyperactivity-impulsivity have persisted for at least 6 months, and are maladaptive and inconsistent compared to people your age.

Hyperactivity

____(a) often fidgets with hands or feet or squirms in seat

____(b) leaves seat in classroom or in other situations in which remaining seated is expected

____(c) often runs about or climbs excessively in situations where it is inappropriate (in adolescents or adults, may be limited to subjective feelings of restlessness)

____(d) often has difficulty playing or engaging in leisure activities quietly

____(e) is often "on the go" or often acts as if "driven by a motor"

____(f) often talks excessively

Impulsivity

____(g) often blurts out answers to questions before the questions have been completed

____(h) often has difficulty waiting in lines or awaiting turn in games or group situations

____(i) often interrupts or intrudes on others

Reprinted with permission from the Diagnostic and Statistical Manual of Mental Disorders, Fourth Edition. Copyright © 1994 American Psychiatric Association.

According to the *DSM-IV,* in order for the above symptoms to qualify you as having ADD, they must (a) have existed since before the age of seven; (b) be present in two or more situations, such as school, work, or home; and (c) not occur as a result of some other disorder.

Based on the foregoing criteria, the *DSM-IV* considers individuals to be the predominantly *Inattentive Type* of AD/HD if six or more of those criteria in section 1 have been met for the past six months; individuals are the predominantly *Hyperactive-Impulsive Type* if six or more of those criteria in section 2 are met. If six or more criteria in *each* category are met, then the individual is the *Combined Type*.

You have probably noticed the lines to the left of each of the AD/HD or ADD symptoms listed here. For each of these symptoms, rate yourself on the following scale:

0 = This problem does not occur in my life, or so little that it doesn't matter.
1 = The problem occurs sometimes and is relatively mild.
2 = The problem occurs at a moderate level, enough to be a problem in my life.
3 = This problem is significant and gets in the way of my life a lot.

Rate yourself on how you are doing at present and score each of the symptoms. This will be your *baseline* score. As you work on various suggestions in this book and try different treatments or medication, you can rate yourself again. If your score is lower, it might be an indication that the treatment is working. We have provided a convenient chart in Appendix A so that you can score yourself at different times, and you can check to see if your scores are lower over time. This scoring system is actually similar (but not identical) to one used by Russell Barkley, a respected researcher in the field (Barkley, 1990, p. 627).

On the list of symptoms circle all scores that you have rated either 2 or 3. Count the items in each of the two categories—*Inattention* and *Hyperactivity-Impulsivity*—and list the *number* of circled items in the first column below. The second column lists the total number of points in each category. Enter your score here, adding up the points in each category:

	NUMBER OF ITEMS SCORED AS 2 OR 3	TOTAL POINTS
Inattention	_____	_____
Hyperactivity- Impulsivity	_____	_____
Total	_____	_____

When you complete this scoring, you have a score on (a) the *number of items* that were selected; and (b) a rough measure of the *severity of each category*. If you have six or more items listed under Inattention, then you qualify as the Inattentive Type of AD/HD. If you have six or more of any of the Hyperactive and Impulsive symptoms, then you qualify as the Hyperactive-Impulsive Type. If you score six or more in each category, you are the Combined Type.

It's also important to keep in mind that there are mental health professionals who believe that ADD is a "made up" problem. So before undergoing expensive testing and evaluation, you should ask the clinician if ADD is a "real" problem for some people. If you get a "no" answer or you are told that it is "extremely rare," then it is likely that you will not be diagnosed with attention deficit disorder—whether you have it or not.

On the other hand it is not necessary for you to see a clinician who only or primarily treats ADD because of the potential pitfall that the mental health professional could see ADD in everyone, when in fact your problem could be a different one. Rather, it's best to see an expert who is knowledgeable and willing to learn about ADD but who is not fixated on attention deficit disorder and treats other problems as well.

This discussion pertains to the official ADD diagnosis given in the *DSM-IV*. Its categories of symptoms and types can raise various issues; and indeed researchers are forever debating the merits of different systems of categorizing disorders. Of course this kind of professional discourse is what pushes the field ahead and also generates new research.

There are other ways we can think about diagnosing the adult with ADD, and some of these alternate theories will be discussed later. These schema are not meant to substitute for the "official" diagnostic criteria but, instead, raise certain important issues that are not raised by the official diagnosis. This is because the history of ADD (and its other labels throughout the last century) mostly has to do with children.

Thus all the ADD definitions—up until the latest edition of the *DSM-IV*—were mainly understood in terms of the problems of childhood. Yet there are certain problems that children do not face with any degree of frequency until their teen years and that are crucially important to adult life. Some key examples are starting and finishing long-term projects, such as completing a college degree; writing a paper for school or a book; picking up the subtle interpersonal cues that let an adult know that a discussion should be postponed; cutting someone off too many times and not noticing the negative impact; planning and organizing a project that has many different components; or dealing with multiple bits of information at one time, as at a business meeting or dinner party. Try to notice when such challenging events come up in your own life as you focus on whether or not you have ADD.

Now let's turn to other aspects of the diagnostic process that play a part in determining if you have ADD.

Medical Screening

It's a good idea for you to be screened by a medical expert such as an internist, neurologist, or psychiatrist who is knowledgeable about ADD and other medical problems. Some medical conditions may resemble ADD but require very different treatment. For example, if you have a problem with an under- or over-active thyroid, it will not be resolved by counseling or taking Ritalin; instead you need medical treatment that will deal with this condition.

Therefore, it's a good idea to see your doctor for a complete workup, including screening for thyroid disease and other common ailments that may be masked as ADD.

Depression or learning disabilities (discussed later in this chapter) may also look like attentional problems. Sometimes a person is born with a problem that makes it difficult for him to process information quickly and accurately. And sometimes a person may have very small seizures, called *petit mal seizures* or *absences,* which may require an electroencephalogram (EEG) to detect. (Sometimes even this test does not pick up the evidence.)

Not all clinicians have the ability to diagnose the rather wide range of problems that may present as ADD. So remember that you must first of all make up your mind, whatever your condition, *never to give up.*

And, second, you must act as your own advocate. This means that even if a person who holds many degrees does not believe that you have ADD (or some other condition), learn more about it anyway. Try new strategies and get the help you need.

Psychological Testing

Many mental health professionals use a variety of psychological tests to help determine if a person has ADD. For example, an intelligence test is frequently used in order to specify various cognitive abilities. It is not because people above or below a certain IQ have ADD.

An intelligence test, such as the Wechsler Adult Intelligence Scale—Revised (WAIS-R), is helpful because the clinician, after determining your level of intelligence, can then look at how you are doing in your life and see if that seems to correlate. Also these scores are compared to other cognitive functions to see if some abilities relating to attention are significantly lower than your level of intelligence.

For example, if you have an IQ of 140, which is at the highest level of intelligence, but you are working as a clerk in a convenience store at age thirty, one might wonder, "What's wrong with this picture?" (Of course, there is nothing wrong with working in a convenience store, and other factors may have led you to that job, such as high unemployment.)

Another factor for the psychologist to consider is whether or not there is a very wide disparity between your verbal IQ score and your performance IQ score. If there is such a disparity—for example, a twenty-or-more-point difference—it is a possible indicator of ADD.

Learning Disabilities

There are other reasons for doing a full battery of psychological tests, such as measuring your various cognitive abilities. For instance, there is a fairly strong connection between ADD and learning disabilities. Anywhere from 40 to 80 percent of people with ADD have a learning disability, according to Larry Silver, M.D., a recognized expert on ADD.

Many laypeople (and some doctors) think that learning disorders and ADD are almost identical. Not true! A learning disorder is defined as some learning function that is significantly below your overall level of intelligence.

For example, if you are very smart but you read slowly, you may have a learning disability in reading speed. Or if, despite scoring at an average level of intelligence, you have a very hard time calculating numbers or balancing your checkbook, it may mean that you have a learning disability in mathematical calculation.

In fact, you could have a learning disability in almost any conceivable cognitive area, including left-right-direction, memory, hearing sounds accurately, hand-writing, foreign languages, spelling, and sounding out words properly, among others.

This is important to note in a book on ADD because sometimes what can appear as an attention problem could actually be a learning problem. As a professional who has been evaluating learning disabilities for about twenty years, I can assure you that tests for learning disabilities take plenty of time—about seven to ten hours of testing and then three to five hours to write the report. As a result, the cost can be about $1,500.

But what the person receives is a precise profile of his or her cognitive abilities. Sometimes for the first time in his life, a person can find out how intelligent he is as well as his level of learning abilities compared with that of other people of the same age.

Sometimes awareness of a previously unrecognized learning disability will be a real eye-opener, and will clarify issues that were previously misunderstood. This actually happened to me.

About ten years ago, I purchased an elaborate test battery for my practice and decided to test myself before I knew the answers. Then, when I read the profile, I said to myself, "My goodness, I have a learning disability!" And then it hit me. Yes, I had always been a slow reader and had had a hard time keeping up with some professors. I would also fall asleep after reading for twenty minutes. And I am left-handed—often a tip-off for learning disabilities. Ever since then, I've had deep sympathy for adults with learning disabilities and ADD, because in some way I know what it is like from the inside.

If a person had a hard time learning in class and yet appears quite intelligent, the problem may not be attention deficit disorder but rather an undiagnosed learning disability. It may be that she has trouble not with attention but with processing information or learning. But this does not have to be an either-or situation. A person may have *both* a learning disorder and ADD. In fact, people with ADD have about a 50 percent likelihood of also having a learning disability.

How Is ADD Different from Depression?

As we have mentioned, other diagnoses can sometimes look like ADD. A depressed person, for example, may have problems paying attention *and* be very distractible. In addition, he or she may be disorganized, having serious problems with time management, procrastination, inability to work in a noisy environment, and irritability with people. These are some of the symptoms of people with ADD as well.

The simplest way to tell if you have ADD is this: Examine your history and see if there is any evidence of ADD in your childhood—hyperactivity, being distractible, not paying attention, forgetting, losing things, or any of the other behaviors we have mentioned. You might find that you need some professional help in order to ferret out these morsels of your history. If these elements of ADD are not part of your life, and if you believe you are depressed, then it is a good idea to seek help for what may be depression.

There is some degree of co-morbidity between ADD and depression. This makes perfect sense, because if the ADD person is not able to complete projects because of problems with attention, and cannot maintain friendships because of the lack of social skills, depression logically follows. If he or she were not depressed, I would wonder!

There is another fact that is important to recognize: For some reason that scientists don't fully understand, some antidepressant medications work well for many ADD patients. It may be that some types of ADD and depression show similar brain chemistries. Or it may be that some action in the brain of the ADD person just happens to be triggered by certain medication and that it has been discovered, by trial and error, by observant doctors.

This sometimes happens in the history of medicine. A certain compound is designed to cure one disorder, and some clever doctor tries the same potion for another condition, observing the effects carefully—and the patient is cured of a problem that no one thought could be cured. The history of medicine is full of such stories—including the discovery of medications that help people with schizophrenia, a serious mental illness; it was found that antihistamines helped to reduce their psychotic thinking.

That is why it is good to be open-minded when you learn about different treatments for ADD, or for other problems that you may confront in learning about your ADD. Bring your new awareness to others whom you encounter on your journey of understanding. Someone may benefit from your knowledge and support.

Other Psychological Tests

The psychologist or psychiatrist may also administer such psychological tests as the Beck Depression Inventory, a commonly used test for depression. This test is good because people often confuse depression with ADD. Of course, you may suffer from both ADD and depression. What the mental health professional needs to determine is: What is the main problem?

Some clinicians use tests such as the Rorschach—the famous ink-blot test. You will be asked what you see in each ink blot, and then the psychologist scores the answers according to an elaborate system that takes quite a while to learn. This test, however, should only be used in conjunction with other tools available to mental health professionals. (A full discussion of many psychological tests and other personality measures is beyond the scope of this book.)

The psychologist may also test you for academic achievement. For example, the Wide Range Achievement Test—Revised (WRAT-R) measures the person's ability to read single words, do pencil-and-paper arithmetic, and spelling. Comparing these scores with a person's intelligence levels can help determine whether or not there is a learning disability.

If a thorough battery of achievement tests is given to determine learning problems, many other abilities are also assessed, including reading comprehension, reading speed, and some of the underlying cognitive processes. A commonly used battery, composed of many tests and used for both children and adults, is the Woodcock Johnson Psycho-Educational Battery.

If a more elaborate neuropsychological evaluation is done, other sets of tests can be used. The two most common batteries are the Halstead-Reitan Battery and the Luria-Nebraska Battery. But many neuropsychologists give other tests.

Additionally, memory tests may also be employed, such as the Selective Reminding Test, the Wechsler Memory Scale, or the Rey-Osterreith Complex Figure Test. These and many other neuropsychological tests are designed to show how well the brain is functioning.

Although such testing is valuable and provides important information, testing alone does not determine an ADD diagnosis. One reason is that people with ADD (including children) can sometimes function very well under structured situations; and testing is just such a situation. So although George has a devil of a time completing his report on marketing for the boss, he can sit for hours surfing the Internet.

Does George really have ADD? And why does he do so well on psychological tests? The answer is that in structured situations smart people with ADD can often do very well. They can temporarily lock themselves into a problem-solving mode. But let them loose in an unstructured situation and they will fall apart.

So what good is all this testing? It provides key pieces of the puzzle needed to make a diagnosis. Let's look at some high-tech tests as well.

Continuous Performance Tests: Using Computer Technology to Assess ADD

Computers can perform some functions that are difficult or impossible for ordinary humans. For example, a computer can track data much more precisely and can measure small amounts of time (such as milliseconds) with far more accuracy than a person could. The computer can also compare scores with those of a normative population, which means it can compare your scores with those of 100 or 1,000 people who are the same age.

Imagine a screen that flashes different images and asks the test taker to push a button if two 5s are followed by an odd number. To perform this task, you must pay attention to the images in front of you and also keep in mind what happened a few seconds ago. So you are asked to keep a few things in your mind at once.

Imagine doing this fifty to a hundred times and under all sorts of conditions. This is the essence of a continuous performance test (CPT). Such a task can be very difficult for a person with ADD. And often they will do poorly on these tests—or so you would think.

Now imagine that instead of just visual images you ask the person to keep in mind information that they hear. This would be called an *auditory* continuous performance test.

Several companies make CPTs, and each claims that theirs is the best. These tests cost about $500, and some companies charge a fee every time the test is used. If a psychologist does use a CPT test on a regular basis, it is a good indicator that he or she is actively involved in treating ADD. However, these tests have drawbacks as well as great potential.

Some Thoughts on CPTs

One problem with continuous performance tests is that they were developed primarily for use with ADD children. Thus their database is usually heavily weighted to a younger population. As a person grows older, cognitive abilities change and mature, so the response of an eight-year-old hyperactive child cannot be presumed to be similar to the reaction time and cognitive functioning of an adult.

One powerful value of these tests is in tracking the response to medications over time. This is because some people with ADD don't know they are getting better—as strange as this might seem. Thus the CPT test could be used to determine whether a person shows improvement on the second or third trial of a medication.

The most popular CPTs on the market currently are

the TOVA (from Universal Attention Disorder, Inc., Los Alamitos, California), the Connors CPT (from Multi-Health Systems, North Tonawanda, New York), and the IVA (from Brain Train, Richmond, Virginia).

One advantage of the TOVA is that it has a Macintosh version. An advantage of the IVA is that it uses both auditory and visual stimuli; unfortunately, it requires special hardware, including computer speakers. An advantage of the Connors is that there is no charge for each test that is used. A drawback of all of these tests is that they do not actually diagnose ADD. But they are good ways to see if medication is working.

Your mental health professional may or may not use this software to assist with diagnosis. It's also likely that as the state of the art advances, other software and hardware products to help diagnose ADD will be developed further. At present, however, not enough research has been completed and published in professional journals to support their utility.

There are other reasons to suggest that CPTs are not yet useful. First, the norms for adults are not generally well developed. For psychiatric tests to be valid, the number of subjects should be 30–80 in each age range. In general, these tests do not have enough of a sample for a sturdy database.

Another issue is validity. What does it mean that someone can respond to fine levels of flashing stimuli? It has not yet been demonstrated clearly in the research that these millisecond measurements are related to important issues in life.

It is likely that as the research is developed, these tests will prove valuable in distinguishing different types of ADD. Even more important, CPTs might be able to predict what medications should be the first to try with different types of ADD. As research data are collected and issues of database and validity are resolved, we may eventually have continuous performance tests that can make treatment far more efficient than it is at present.

Personal History

According to most professionals in the field, a person's history is the most important factor in diagnosing ADD. Some professionals say that ADD is diagnosed by history, not by test. Strictly speaking, this is true, since the definition of ADD at present has to do with overt symptoms that a person reports about his or her life, both in the past and in the present.

In fact, if you want a very simple way to diagnose ADD, you can rate yourself on the *DSM-IV* symptoms as you did earlier in the chapter, but first rate yourself as you were when you were a child. Then do another rating, assessing yourself as you are now.

If you had ADD as a child, you are a likely candidate for being an ADD adult. Now put your scores from childhood next to the scores you obtained as an adult and compare the two. How much has your ADD persisted into adulthood?

Scores on Self-Rating Tests (in Chapter 1)

SCALE	AS A CHILD	AS A TEENAGER	AS AN ADULT
Inattention	_____	_____	_____
Hyperactivity-Impulsivity	_____	_____	_____
Total	_____	_____	_____

Taking a personal history in some detail, therefore, is going to be one of the first things the clinician will do, so it's a good idea to put together in your mind various facts and stories that illustrate what you were like as a child.

What was your mood as a child? How did you do in school? Did you have many friends or were you a loner? Did you get into fights, steal things, or do daring acts for a thrill? Go over the list of symptoms again and really give this some thought.

Because it may be very hard for you to present a true picture of your childhood—since most people's impressions of childhood become distorted as they grow older—the mental health professional may also wish to talk with family members or your parents with your permission.

The psychologist may also suggest that you ask your relatives certain questions and bring this information to your next session. You may even be asked to seek out old report cards to see if there are any clues to the possibility of childhood ADD.

Of course, your adult life is important, too, and the psychologist may ask if you are married, if you are employed, how many times you've been married, how many jobs you've had, and other questions.

How you feel now is important because the psychologist is trying to determine how debilitating the ADD is for you. Do you feel that you are being held back, and do you feel like you really have problems with attention, distractibility, and organization? Do you want to change? This is also an important factor, since many times in therapy a person may say he wants to change, but will not put in the effort needed to make his life better. The psychologist can't wave a magic wand and make you "all better." There's plenty of work for you to do as well. But the psychologist can help you by serving as a guide or coach as you try to improve your life circumstances.

The Chronic Nature of Your Problem

Another key factor is the length of time your symptoms have been a problem for you. Has it been a few months, a few years, or most of your life? If you have been coping effectively for most of your adult life and are suddenly having serious difficulty managing, the problem could be something other than ADD and can be explored with an experienced clinician.

A key feature of ADD is its chronicity: That means it's not a new problem but one that you've been struggling with for years. As a result, if your procrastination, distractibility, disorganization, and other symptoms appear to be new issues for you, it's less likely that you have ADD.

On the other hand, you may have had ADD for a long time, but it may not have been a problem because of your high intelligence level, good environment, and other factors. Some important circumstance may have changed in your life and triggered the problem—or made it emerge, even though it was always there. You may have encountered a change in jobs, stressful life events, or other problems, and reached the limit of your ability to cope—somewhat like a glass being filled to the brim and then spilling over. The mental health professional should take this possibility into account as well.

Self-Ratings

The clinician may ask you to rate yourself on a scale of questions, either one that he or she has devised or one that is generally accepted as a good tool. For example, the rating devices offered in Chapter 1 and in this chapter could be helpful.

Other Theories of Adult ADD

There are several other ways of thinking about ADD that can help you deepen your understanding and view your condition in a more flexible way. The theories are identified with their authors, who I discuss in this chapter. You can learn more about them by consulting the back of the book for a list of recommended books and other resources offered by experts on ADD.

Paul Wender, M.D.

Paul Wender, a psychiatrist, is a pioneer in the field of attention deficit disorder. He initially studied children; but as the years passed, he began to see some of these children as adults, and they were still having problems. Many of them had symptoms of ADD, but these were somewhat different from the symptoms they had as children. Wender and his colleagues have developed the Utah Criteria for adult ADD. These guidelines are slightly different from the official *DSM-IV* criteria, and they require the adult to have had *hyperactivity* as a child and to *continue* to manifest hyperactivity in some way. By hyperactivity, Wender means some kind of persistent motor activity—which we can think of as restlessness obvious enough to be physical—as well as attention deficits. One must also manifest two of the following five symptoms: emotional instability, inability to complete tasks, hot temper, impulsivity, and intolerance of stress. In addition, adults must not have other major psychiatric disorders that might explain their symptoms. This set of criteria has not been universally accepted by professionals; one reason is that it leaves out the ADD type that does not show hyperactivity, the Inattentive Type (Murphy, 1995; Lahey and Carlson, 1991; DSM-IV, 1994).

Because Wender is a major figure in the field, his symptom criteria are given serious attention by professionals. His recent book on adult attention deficit disorder (see "Recommended Books") is written for the professional and is very technical. But it is probably one of the best books that describes the various studies that have been done with respect to etiology, or the causes of ADD.

Russell Barkley, Ph.D.

Russell Barkley is one of the most respected ADD researchers, and he, too, has spent most of his career studying children. (He is also an excellent speaker and worth going out of your way to hear.) Barkley believes that ADD without hyperactivity is a disorder *separate* from the types of ADD that include hyperactivity (Barkley, 1990). He understands ADD as a disorder of the ability to inhibit, or hold back, responses—which would include the ability to delay a response. By considering this as the main problem, Barkley believes he can better explain the typical adult ADD problems, such as poor time management, the inability to pursue goals consistently, failing to pay attention to social cues (because of behaving impulsively and missing the cues), and the inability to plan. Even if Barkley turns out to be correct that ADD without hyperactivity is a separate disorder, the attention problems still exist and merit professional treatment.

Thomas E. Brown, Ph.D.

Thomas E. Brown is a psychologist with some interesting ways of thinking about ADD in adults. He proposes an "expanded model" of ADD in adults (Brown, 1995) that highlights the following five clusters of problems:

1. *Activating and organizing*—which includes difficulty getting started and organized for work and daily routines
2. *Sustaining attention*—particularly with work tasks, which might include daydreaming or distractibility when reading or listening
3. *Sustaining energy and effort*—especially for work tasks, which can result in daytime sleepiness and slacking off except when the pressure is on
4. *Moodiness and sensitivity to criticism*—including irritability and apparent lack of motivation
5. *Memory recall*—problems remembering names, dates, or material necessary for work

Dr. Brown has noted that many hyperactive children become adults who have ADD *without* hyperactivity, or the Inattentive Type. Of course, this is one of the principal reasons why ADD appears to go away as the person grows older: The outward signs are gone, but the inner inattentiveness remains—and is often misunderstood.

Edward Hallowell, M.D., and John Ratey, M.D.

Doctors Hallowell and Ratey are the authors of *Driven to Distraction,* a well-written and important book about adult ADD. Since they have treated adults for a number of years, they have discovered ways of describing the special features of adults with ADD, in contrast to the view of adult symptoms as muted versions of childhood symptoms. And they suggest criteria, such as the following, for diagnosing adult ADD that are different from, and additional to, those listed in *DSM-IV:*

- A chronic sense of underachievement
- Problems getting organized
- Impulsivity, both verbally and behaviorally, as in changing career plans, sudden trips, spending money
- Intolerance of boredom
- Tendency to worry too much
- A sense of insecurity, low self-esteem
- Chronic procrastination
- Tendency to be creative and highly intuitive
- Tendency to have many simultaneous projects
- Mood swings
- Tendency toward addictive behaviors
- Inaccurate perception of self

Thom Hartmann

Thom Hartmann is *not* a psychiatrist or psychologist, as are the people I have just discussed. He is the father of an ADD child and operated a treatment facility for children. After his son was diagnosed with ADD, he began to think about how society seemed to stereotype these children as negative or maladjusted.

According to his theory, in prehistoric times *hunters* killed animals for food and brought these prizes back to the rest of the clan. The hunter had the ability to notice small movements in the brush, to act immediately in order to kill the animal or defend himself, along with other traits that we might today categorize as impulsive or hyperactive. Long ago, these same skills were not only adaptive but highly valued. Then society changed into an agricultural system in which the *farmer's* traits were valued—patient, careful, plodding day by day, a steady type.

In Hartmann's view, the ADD person is like the hunter, out of place in today's society of farmers. In developing his ideas, Hartmann discovered that entrepreneurs often seemed to resemble ADD people: They are the ones who take risks, who are independent, who are aware of details that others miss (hyperactivity?). They enjoy the "hunt," and they are results oriented.

One of the most important aspects of his theory is that it reframes the ADD person in a positive light and in some ways empowers the person. But there are some drawbacks: It does not adequately take into account that the ADD person often suffers and *wants* to become less distracted and more effective in managing life. His book is worth reading, if only because of its way of viewing the "negative" qualities of ADD as "positive" ones.

The James Lawrence Thomas Method: The Simplest Way to Know if You Have Adult ADD

Please answer the following questions:

1. Do your attention problems (such as distractibility or forgetting) get in the way of your life?_____

2. Has this been true since you were very young (prior to age seven)?_____

If you answered·yes to both of these questions, it is possible (but not confirmed) that you have attention deficit disorder. This assumes that there are no other psychological problems that may better explain your condition. And that is why you need to consult a professional. You also need to see a professional because no one (including myself) can objectively define his or her personal situation. Having the support and guidance of that outside person is important. If a therapist or clinician has an understanding of adult ADD, then he or she can be especially helpful in working on the issues you need to resolve.

It is my own personal belief that you could have ADD even if you answer only the first question with a yes. There are several ways to think about it. First, you may not have been diagnosed as a child. Second, you may be the nonhyperactive type, who, not fitting the classic ADD profile, was not diagnosed. Third, the ADD may not have been manifested in early childhood because you did not then have to exercise the higher-level attentional skills involved in completing complex projects or learning vast amounts of difficult material—as in medical board exams, for example. Fourth, I propose the possibility of a later onset of ADD because of factors such as substance abuse, a particularly demanding career choice (such as law or medicine), subtle learning disabilities, or a mild head injury. Note that this view of an adult onset of ADD is not held by most professionals in the field; it is my hypothesis and may be clarified by future research.

Is ADD Overdiagnosed?

After having considered the ADD diagnosis and other ways to think about the disorder, what about the claim that ADD in adults is a lot of hype, simply the latest trendy diagnosis—what the media calls the diagnosis of the nineties. Everywhere you look, people are being diagnosed with ADD.

Just because it is talked about a great deal does not make the diagnosis illegitimate. Anyone who has experienced being in the presence of a truly hyperactive child knows that such a child is not like other children. Recent evidence of some differences in ADD brain chemistry has been presented. And the volumes of research on ADD children should be able to convince most people that ADD is a real disorder. If, in fact, children are overdiagnosed, that may have more to do with other factors, such as the need for children to be cooperative in their crowded classrooms or the fact that, in many households, both parents are working and have less time for their active, playful, or frustrated children. This issue awaits detailed research. We have considered the reasons why many professionals believed that children outgrew ADD, and why the nonhyperactive type of ADD is now accepted. Given the fact that the most obvious childhood expressions of ADD are muted in later years, it is not surprising that many ADD children continue to have symptoms when they grow up.

The best validation is to look at your own experience—or that of someone you know. Have you gained a new understanding of your problems by considering ADD as the underlying cause? Those of you who have suffered from ADD in adulthood can testify that your lives have been compromised—by chronic disorganization, lateness for appointments, failure to complete work projects, frequently getting fired from jobs, or otherwise not living up to your potential. The same can be said to a great extent for adults who have a learning disability.

Russell Barkley, a leader in the field of ADD, has noted that the increased awareness of the disorder has led to an increase in the number of referrals. But only careful, precise research will enable us to know in the long run to what extent ADD has been overdiagnosed.

Perhaps it is overdiagnosed. But it is just as likely that it is underdiagnosed. Maybe too many people—especially children—are given Ritalin in an effort to make them more cooperative. But it may also be the case that many adults who are currently treated for depression or other disorders would be better off if they were viewed as adults with ADD.

Conclusion

Although ADD can be difficult for even an experienced clinician to diagnose, experts know what signposts to look out for. However, professionals are limited by what you tell them—background information and personal history, and some test results that can help distinguish between ADD and other conditions. The diagnostic information on ADD, especially in an adult, is not perfect. But as researchers gain more information, and as you persist in self-education, you will have a better sense of where you stand.

6

Treating ADD with Medication

"My medication helps me to concentrate for long periods of time and stick to one subject. In fact, it was actually upsetting for me to realize how much it really helped me—it made this disorder seem worse!" said Molly, who has found considerable relief from her ADD symptoms by taking Dexedrine spansules. (Spansules are timed-release medications. Dexedrine spansules last eight to twelve hours.)

Ted, a man who takes Ritalin, the most frequently prescribed medication for ADD, observed, "I feel like Ritalin gives me a focusing ability I never had before. And it helped my moods too. When I first started taking Ritalin, I didn't feel frustrated all the time and I wasn't as moody. My wife noticed it more even than I did—she calls it my Happy Pill. It doesn't really make me feel happy, but when you're not frustrated all the time about little things, you feel happy."

Many adults diagnosed with ADD take medication, which is often the same as that used by children and adolescents with ADD. Medications don't "cure" ADD, but they can alleviate the symptoms significantly. As a result, the person experiences a sense of empowerment in dealing with the problems of disorganization, distractibility, and other hallmark features of ADD.

It is important to keep in mind, however, that no medication can completely eradicate these problems. You will still need to make a conscious choice—and to work—to effect changes in your life. Effective medications can give you an edge, a kind of leg up over the stone wall of untreated ADD. Psychiatrist Paul Wender has said that when medications work, it's like giving vitamin C to a person with scurvy. It's what they most need to resolve the problem.

One very frustrating problem of treating ADD with medication is that it is often a trial-and-error process. Your doctor chooses one medication for you, sees if it helps, questions you about it, and then adjusts dosages or changes the medication altogether.

Rarely are there quick fixes with ADD medications. And even if a medication works for you, you still have to face the ups and downs of daily life. It's also true that medications sometimes lose their efficacy, and your physician may have to switch you to another drug or change the dose. What is likely to be different for you (when the medication works) is that your ups and downs will more closely resemble the ups and downs of a person who does not have ADD. So you essentially level the playing field of life.

Some medications are long-lasting (for eight to twelve hours or more), while others last only two to four hours. In some cases, physicians combine long-lasting and short-acting medications. For example, a typical strategy is to prescribe a short-acting medication in the afternoon in order to continue the positive effects of the stimulant but forgo possible problems with insomnia and other side effects that could be caused by a second long-acting dose.

This chapter provides a general overview of the key medications used today in treating ADD and also discusses some of the problems in prescribing and taking these medications. It's important to understand that this chapter is only a guide and that it is ultimately up to your doctor—not you—to decide which medications are appropriate.

Before Medication Many Self-Medicate

Experts hypothesize that adults with ADD sometimes unconsciously attempt to medicate themselves with large amounts of caffeine, in the form of coffee or colas. "I took huge amounts of caffeine without realizing why," says Larry, who is now being treated with Ritalin. He says his caffeine craving has been greatly reduced—probably because the brain biochemistry is somehow adjusted.

Sometimes medications taken for hay fever seem to help, and people who don't realize they have ADD notice that antihistamines seem to help them focus better. However, such medications can be dangerous on top of stimulants or other ADD medications.

Sadly, some adults self-medicate with alcohol or illegal substances such as cocaine. The ADDer may notice that cocaine makes him think rationally while his friends who don't have ADD become euphoric under the influence of this dangerous drug.

Tracking Your Own Reactions Is Important

In deciding what medications to use, physicians must rely very heavily on patients' self-reports to determine whether a medication is effective or not. There are no blood or urine tests that can determine if you are receiving the optimal level of an ADD medication, and even sophisticated technology such as PET scans cannot determine the dosage level that is right for you.

As a result, your doctor will ask you to note how you are feeling within hours or days of taking a medication and to report that information later. Some medications, such as Ritalin, act in the body immediately, while others, such as Zoloft, have a cumulative effect, which you won't feel fully for weeks.

Remember, in the introduction to this book, when I asked you to keep track of certain behaviors that could be indicators of whether or not you are improved? I called these *behavioral markers*. Such behaviors can be small and insignificant, or they could be more substantial. But they should be viewed as behaviors that may indicate—if they improve—that you are better. That is, they *mark* your progress.

This is a way to get an independent handle on how you are doing. You would systematically keep track of these behaviors in order to observe how they are affected by different treatment interventions. This might even help make your treatment more efficient. Yet, I will be the first one to admit that tracking this kind of data is often very hard for people with ADD because they are not used to recording *anything* in a systematic way. But do try.

For example, if one of your behavioral markers is losing things, and you note as you keep track of this behavior that you lose things less and less each week, then you are getting better. If you start losing things more frequently, you are getting worse.

How do you know what your behavioral markers are? You look at patterns of behavior that differ when you are effective from when you are not. Make a two-column list. Label one column *Well* and the other column *Problem.* Think about how your behavior differs from one state to another.

Ask your spouse or significant other and family members what things you do when your ADD symptoms are more severe. Do you yell more? Do you drop things? Do you have a messier or clean(er) desk? Once you determine your own personal behavioral markers, you can better evaluate how you're doing *and* report this information to your therapist.

Rating Yourself

The doctor or therapist may also zero in on primary problems such as inattentiveness, moodiness, or other symptoms and ask you to rate yourself on a weekly basis, perhaps using a scale for this purpose—for example, 10 for much worse, 5 for about the same, 3 for better, and 1 for much better.

However, a common problem among people with ADD is that they forget to rate themselves. Or, if they do the ratings, they forget to bring them in to the doctor. Still, it's important to make that effort because the doctor really does need your feedback to determine whether or not to adjust dosages or change the medication altogether.

If you do need to change your medication, follow

your doctor's instructions to the letter. It's a good idea to take notes, so bring along a small pad of paper when you go to the doctor. Many ADDers find that if they write things down, they remember them better. Of course, you must make an effort not to lose your notes or your notebook.

Medications Can Have Temporary (or Long-Lasting) Side Effects

Another factor to keep in mind is that sometimes a medication may give you some temporary discomforting side effects—such as sweating, nausea, or other side effects that your doctor will (or should) tell you about—but your body will often adjust. Be sure to ask your doctor if there are any serious side effects that you should watch out for—for example elevated blood pressure when you are taking a stimulant medication.

Sometimes the doctor may prescribe another medication to resolve the problems caused by the ADD medication, but that isn't always possible. If the side effects are intolerable, be sure to tell your doctor so that another medication can be considered.

You may wish to ask your doctor if you can start the new medication over the weekend so that any possible discomfort or side effects won't interfere with your work. You may be able to overcome (or at least lessen) any side effects by the time Monday rolls around.

Most Physicians Start Slowly with Medication

Generally, physicians start patients on the lowest possible dose of a medication. If it later seems indicated or necessary, they will increase the dosage in the light of a dosage limit that they will not go beyond. It's interesting to note that the dosage level does not correlate to your weight; and some physicians have said that small children sometimes require a larger dosage than bigger children. Presumably, this also holds true for adults.

Your physician may ultimately choose to use several different medications simultaneously to treat your ADD. However, usually only one medication is added at a time so that the doctor may determine which medication is doing what. For example, the doctor may choose to prescribe both a stimulant, such as Ritalin, and an antidepressant, such as Norpramine. Most physicians may start with the stimulant and later add the antidepressant. Others, such as Dr. John Ratey, start with Norpramine, then add the stimulant.

In addition, your doctor (or you) may choose to contact experts in the field. For example, in 1994 pharmacist Peter Anderson formed Med-ADD Services in Boston, Massachusetts, a consulting company that specializes in advising on medications for attention deficit disorder. Anderson also publishes a newsletter dealing with ADD medications.

Generally, however, physicians rely on published journal articles, their own experience, and the experiences of respected colleagues to determine what medications and what dosages to prescribe for their ADD patients.

Consult a Doctor Experienced in Treating Adult ADD

Keep in mind that only a medical doctor can prescribe medication; and for this reason, many adults with ADD consult a psychiatrist, neurologist, or general practitioner. Your doctor should have experience in treating adult ADD. (See Chapter 7 for information on identifying a good doctor.) In general, you want a psychiatrist who specializes in trying out different medications. They are sometimes called psychopharmacologists.

It is true that a few adults have obtained their prescriptions from their child's pediatrician or their own former pediatrician because they say it's hard to find a psychiatrist who will treat them. Other adults have convinced physicians from other states to prescribe medications for them. In my opinion, this is recommended only if you cannot find someone local.

You need to consult with a physician who will follow your case and who can actually see you on an as-needed basis. Telephone consultations are helpful and convenient, but these alone are not the best way to work with a doctor. Those of you who live in more remote areas of the country may not have a choice, however.

You might also collect articles and help educate your local physician, assuming the doctor is open-minded enough to accept what you have to offer.

Fear of Prescribing Stimulants Still Exists

One additional problem faced by many adults with ADD is that some physicians are still hesitant to prescribe stimulant medications, primarily because of the abuse of amphetamines and other stimulants that sometimes occurs. And if the doctor prescribes such a medication, patients have reported difficulties with some pharmacists.

These problems seem to be decreasing, however, as medical and pharmaceutical professionals become more knowledgeable about adult ADD. The medications of choice, as described in this chapter, are known as part of the typical treatment for adult ADD. So there is some scientific research to support you. But keep in mind that some doctors still have old prejudices.

If you have ever had a problem with alcohol or drug abuse, physicians are particularly loath to prescribe a drug such as Dexedrine or Ritalin because they fear you may fall into a pattern of abuse. However, studies so far indicate that abuse is rare among treated ADD adults. The reason is, apparently, that the Dexedrine or Ritalin does not give the ADD person a euphoric high but instead makes him feel normal.

Research on ADD Drugs for Adults Is Scanty but Does Exist

Most researchers have concentrated on the effectiveness of ADD medications for children rather than adults, since only during the past five to ten years have physicians realized that ADD does not end in adolescence. However, an article in the August 1995 issue of the *Journal of Clinical Psychopharmacology* (Wilens et al., 1995) discussed eight studies relating to the effectiveness of stimulants on adults with ADD and eleven studies on the effectiveness of nonstimulant medication. Although the studies were designed differently, and in some cases dosages may have been too low for ADD adults, it was clear that medications could improve symptoms in many adults with ADD.

In a study that looked at the effects of methylphenidate (Ritalin) on adults with ADD, reported in the June 1995 issue of the *Archives of General Psychiatry*, researchers (Spencer et al.) found a very strong therapeutic response to the drug: 78 percent responded to the medication as opposed to 4 percent who responded to the placebo (sugar pill). The reason why researchers believed they found such high response rates was that they dosed the patients according to their weight and up to 1.0 mg/kg per day, which was significantly more than the 0.6 mg/kg used in most other studies.

They found only slight improvements with lower doses and far more dramatic improvements at higher doses. Thus it appears that adults need to receive what researchers call a robust dosage. Of course, the precise dosage—if you are placed on medication—must be determined by your physician. You might suggest that your doctor review this study. Or better yet bring the study in with you!

Stimulant Medications

Stimulant medications are the most frequently prescribed drugs for adults and children with ADD because these drugs seem to help the person concentrate and decrease the distractibility and "spacing out" that is common among ADDers. Brain studies have actually revealed changes in the brain after people have taken a stimulant medication, which lends support to the idea that the medication is helping to correct a chemical imbalance in the brain.

What apparently happens is that the brain of the person with ADD is somewhat sluggish, and as a direct result he or she may become jumpy or inattentive. The stimulants work to provide that extra jolt to the brain and sort of jump-start it into working at a more normal speed.

According to Tim Wilens, M.D., improvement as a result of stimulant medication is most noted in people with the most severe ADD symptoms. There is less improvement in people with a mild form of ADD.

As with any medication, you need to watch out for possible interactions with other medications you take. For example, if you take one of the stimulant medications for ADD, you should avoid decongestants if you get a cold or hay fever: Many cold medicines are also stimulating and you should not overstimulate your brain or body. Certainly you should not take decongestants or antihistamines on a regular basis unless you first clear it with your physician.

Not all psychiatrists choose stimulants as their first line of defense; for example, John Ratey, M.D., a psychiatrist and the coauthor of *Driven to Distraction,* has reported at ADD conferences that he prefers to start his patients on antidepressants. If that is ineffective, he will move to a stimulant medication. Other doctors start immediately with Ritalin or another stimulant once they diagnose a person with ADD.

Ritalin™

The most frequently prescribed medication for both children and adults with ADD is Ritalin, or methylphenidate, which is the generic name. This medication comes in either the brand name (Ritalin) or the generic form. It is also available in a timed-release pill in both the brand name and the generic form. Ritalin takes an hour or two to get into your system and start working (Wilens, Spencer, and Biederman, 1995). Some patients and their physicians would like to see Ritalin in a patch form—like a bandage that you stick on your skin once every few days—so that they'd be less likely to forget the medication. But so far this is not available.

Ritalin is a controlled medication and physicians may prescribe only one month's supply at a time, depending on the state laws. This means that the medication is not automatically refillable.

Some people believe that Ritalin is overcontrolled, and they have lobbied for Ritalin to be moved from a Schedule II drug to a Schedule III (less controlled) medication. This is a very controversial issue right now.

The argument for less control of Ritalin is that it has been shown not to be harmful; in fact, it is one of the safer drugs according to research evidence. The other argument is that Ritalin is still a stimulant drug and has the potential to be misused. So the government, which works very slowly as we all know, would rather err on the safe side than take responsibility for potential negative effects.

Do most adults with ADD respond to Ritalin? Although there is disagreement about the percentage of diagnosed adults who have a favorable response to

Ritalin, depending on which study you look at, it appears that at least half, and as much as nearly 80 percent, of the adults with ADD show a significant and positive response to this medication.

Studies seem to indicate that the lowest dosages are far less effective with adults than higher dosages. But it is important to realize that each person is different. We'd probably all like some magic formula that could let us know just what dose to take. But of course that decision should be left to the prescribing physicians. One person may need a high dose for the medication to work effectively, whereas someone else may require a low dose (Wilens, et al.).

One of my patients takes one quarter of one 5-milligram pill of Ritalin each day; if he takes more than that, he does not do as well. His response to such a low dose is somewhat unusual, but doctors who have experience in medicating patients with adult ADD have probably run into such a patient every once in a while. Such patients may be sensitive to many drugs, even aspirin; this is known as *sensitive brain syndrome*.

Dr. John Ratey tells of patients who use very small amounts of Dexedrine and find that it is plenty for their particular body chemistries.

Some adults need an antidepressant or other medication to supplement their Ritalin. For others, the Ritalin alone works well. And still others report that the Ritalin doesn't work for them at all. It makes them more jittery and nervous and doesn't improve their concentration or their ability to focus. They may also experience insomnia, headaches, and weight loss. So they need to try an alternative medication.

One interesting study of older depressed patients (with an average age of about seventy-two years), reported in the June 1995 issue of the *American Journal of Psychiatry* (Wallace et al., 1995), found that methylphenidate worked well in resolving the depression. It's not clear if this generic form of Ritalin may have an antidepressant effect also on younger people who take it for ADD.

Dexedrine™

Dexedrine (dextroamphetamine) is an amphetamine (known as an upper), and for this reason some physicians and the general public are concerned about its potential abuse. When administered by a trained clinician, there should be no problem. Dexedrine is sometimes an effective medication for treating ADD because it has a "softer" effect on many people. And, at the low dosage typical for ADD treatment, it is not likely to become habit forming.

Like Ritalin, prescriptions for Dexedrine are nonrefillable, so you will need a new one when it's time for a refill. Generally physicians will prescribe Dexedrine for up to thirty days. Dexedrine comes in a tablet as well as a timed-release form. Some people prefer the timed-release capsule because of the convenience and the long-lasting effect.

This means they don't have to remember to take an afternoon pill. It should not surprise you that many adults with ADD have difficulty remembering to take their afternoon medication. Presuming they can remember to take their morning Dexedrine capsule, they're set for about eight to twelve hours.

Be sure to let your doctor know if you have any allergies to cold medicine or other substances, including dyes, foods, or preservatives. The same advice holds true for those of you who may take Ritalin or Cylert. It's also essential that you tell your doctor about other prescribed or over-the-counter medications that you take. Don't presume that if you can buy it yourself in the drugstore, it doesn't count. It does. Also be sure to tell your doctor about your consumption of coffee and tea. Don't forget alcohol consumption: In some cases even a small amount of alcohol could have a negative interaction with your medication and could cause a headache or make you feel sick in some other way.

You should also tell your doctor about any other medical problem, particularly high blood pressure, anxiety, glaucoma, or any serious illness. If you have had a problem with using alcohol or other drugs to excess, be frank with your doctor. Remember, you are trying to make your life better, not put it in jeopardy.

Dexedrine, like all prescription drugs, needs to be taken under the watchful eye of an experienced medical doctor. Therefore, none of the following should be taken as advice on how to take these medications.

Dexedrine comes in single-dosage pills and in timed-release capsules called spansules. The spansules last for about eight to twelve hours and the shorter-acting medications for around four hours. The person who takes Dexedrine should be able to notice fairly quickly (within hours) whether or not the medication has an effect.

Most doctors do not recommend that you take this medication before going to bed, nor should you take the other stimulants before you plan to sleep. If you're taking the shorter-lasting version of Dexedrine, most doctors recommend that you plan to take your last pill at least six hours before bedtime. If you're taking the long-lasting medication, take the last dose as long as ten to fourteen hours *before* you want to sleep.

One problem with Dexedrine, as with Ritalin, is that you may find there is a "rebound effect." This means that when the drug wears off, you are more nervous than before you took the medication—as if your original ADD were temporarily magnified. This problem may actually be worse after taking the short-acting Dexedrine or Ritalin pills as opposed to the timed-release spansules.

Some physicians try to counter the rebound effect by prescribing a lower dose of the drug to take at or near the time when its effect would be wearing off. The rebound effect is apparently much more of a problem in children than it is in adults.

As with Ritalin, Dexedrine may make a person nervous and edgy and may also cause headaches, insomnia, and other side effects. As a result, some people cannot tolerate this medication, although the side effects generally disappear within hours.

Cylert™

Pemoline (Cylert) is another stimulant medication that may work effectively for you. Your doctor can call in a prescription for Cylert, as is not the case with Ritalin or Dexedrine. This is a long-lasting medication that comes in tablets or in chewable form.

Pemoline differs from both Ritalin and Dexedrine in that it does not usually reach its optimal level in the body for at least seven to ten days, or even longer (Wilens, Spencer, and Biederman, 1995). It is often preferred because it is taken in only one dose per day: This is especially convenient for people who forget to take their medicine or for children who might have trouble taking their medication at school.

Antidepressants

Antidepressants are medications that work on the brain to increase the level of primary biochemicals such as dopamine, norepinephrine, or serotonin in your brain.

There are several different categories of antidepressants. Tricyclic antidepressants are traditional medications that have been in use for many years. Selective serotonin reuptake inhibitors, sometimes known as SSRIs, are a newer class of antidepressants: two examples are Prozac and Zoloft. In a different category is Wellbutrin, an atypical antidepressant that has a stimulant effect on the brain. Because of its combined biochemical action, some physicians choose Wellbutrin to treat both ADD and depression. A new antidepressant that may prove to be effective is Effexor.

A different class of antidepressants are the monoamine oxidase inhibitors (MAOIs), such as pargyline and deprenyl. These medications, however, require you to monitor your diet very carefully and thus are generally not the first choice to treat the person with ADD. In fact, they are generally a third or fourth choice (Wilens, Spencer, and Biederman, 1995).

We can expect new antidepressants and other psychiatric medications to become available over the next five to ten years. Experienced and well-qualified physicians will keep themselves up-to-date on which medications are most effective for you.

Tricyclic Antidepressants

Tricyclic antidepressants (TCAs) are often used to treat ADD. Sometimes the TCA is used alone, or it may be used in conjunction with other medications. Little research has been done on adults with ADD who are treated with tricyclics. However, a 1995 research study reported by Wilens and his colleagues in the *Journal of Nervous and Mental Disease* revealed that in adults with ADD who were nonresponsive to stimulants (or for some other reason could not take them) and who experienced other problems such as depression and anxiety, a trial of tricyclics was effective in reducing the ADD symptoms in 68 percent of the adults. Of these, 54 percent were either much improved or very much improved.

Examples of tricyclic antidepressants used to treat adults with ADD are desipramine, nortriptyline, and imipramine. Generally these medications are given at lower dosages than the amount given to a person who suffers from major depression. Side effects of the tricyclics can be dry mouth, constipation, and sleepiness, among others.

Newer Antidepressants

Many people have heard of Prozac, a popular antidepressant in the class of selective serotonin reuptake inhibitors (SSRIs), and one that has received plenty of press, both good and bad. A cousin to Prozac is Zoloft, which some doctors prescribe to treat ADD alone or as a supplement to medications such as Ritalin or Dexedrine. To date, studies have not revealed whether or not Prozac and Zoloft are truly effective in treating adult ADD.

Side effects with SSRIs can include nervousness, insomnia, tiredness, or sexual problems in males, and must be weighed against the benefits that the medication may bring to the patient. Often, however, these side effects may not occur, or they may be mild.

MAO Inhibitors

Another class of antidepressant medications sometimes used to treat ADD are the MAO inhibitors. Some studies have shown moderate improvements in hyperactive children who took medication of this type. Because the patient must follow a strict dietary regimen and avoid certain foods, these medications haven't gained the popularity of the other drugs described in this chapter.

Side effects that have been reported in some people who take this class of drugs are sleepiness, weight gain, and sexual dysfunction.

Wellbutrin™

Wellbutrin (bupropion), an atypical antidepressant, is a stimulating medication that affects the dopamine in the brain. Psychiatrist Paul Wender, author of several books on ADD, has reported success with this medication, although other psychiatrists have been dubious about its efficacy. In one of Wender's studies of nineteen adults, patients improved moderately or markedly in 74 percent of the cases; however, this sample is very small.

The upside of Wellbutrin is that it can work for both ADD and depression. So if a person suffers from both problems, this medication may well be worth a try. The downside is that pills must be taken at least six hours apart because of the potential to cause seizures (Wilens, Spencer, and Biederman, 1995). As a result, most physicians will prescribe the lowest possible dose of this medication and gradually increase it until a favorable response occurs or side effects intervene.

As with all medications, Wellbutrin has side effects, including headache, nausea, weight loss, and other symptoms. The most serious of these is that it may induce seizures in people who are prone to them.

There have also been some reports that Wellbutrin may act as an aphrodisiac; both men and women have noted an increased sex drive while on the medication. This may happen because a previous depression is now resolved, allowing people to look forward to having sex, or for some other reason. In other cases, men have reported a problem with sexual function. And still others remain about the same. As with most medications, individual responses to the drug vary greatly from person to person.

Combinations of Medications

Physicians sometimes combine different medications for a "synergistic" effect: this means that two (or more) medications boost the response more than a single medication. For example, the physician may put you on Ritalin for ADD and Prozac for depression. Or Ritalin and desipramine. Or some other combination of two or more medications, depending on your symptoms and problems.

Off-Label Medications

In some cases, physicians have claimed success in treating ADD with medications typically prescribed for other purposes; that is, they prescribe a drug that has been used primarily to treat another medical problem. For example, the high-blood-pressure drug Tenex (guanfacine) has been used as a supplemental medication to help control aggressiveness and temper tantrums in hyperactive children. It's not clear whether or not this medication would work well on adults with similar symptoms.

Other "antihypertensives" such as clonidine have been used with children and adults who are extremely aggressive and/or hyperactive, although this medication has not been studied on adults with ADD to date. But it is used frequently to decrease the impulsivity in hyperactive people as well as to reduce the tics that sometimes occur with stimulant medication.

Beta-blockers such as propranolol were used in a small sample of adults who were prone to outbursts of temper. But the study results aren't clear-cut because these adults had major behavioral problems and their response may not extend to adults with ADD who are not aggressive (Wilens, Spencer, and Biederman, 1995).

Is It Working?

A feeling of euphoria, no problems, heaven here on earth: If you feel that way after taking one of the medications described in this chapter, something is wrong. The medications should not make you feel blissful or "zoned out"; instead, the goal is to help you skew your chemical imbalance toward normalcy. The best measure of this would be your effectiveness in everyday life, and that's where the behavioral markers come in.

One rather peculiar phenomenon I have noticed over the years of working with ADD adults is that they sometimes do not know when they are getting better. Sounds odd, doesn't it? But they actually have to hear their spouse say, "Oh, yes, you are better, you don't fight so much now. And you do things you didn't do before. I certainly notice the difference!"

Your feelings are also important and should not be neglected. You may feel more in control and better able to concentrate, and that is a sign that the medication is helping you. Or you may feel nothing at all. In fact, many people don't feel much different when taking one of these medications, but they do notice that they're receiving positive (or negative) feedback from spouses, family members, and friends.

Maybe now you can finish that project you've set aside, and you go ahead and do it, not realizing that you started and stopped innumerable times before and just could never get through it. But now you can.

Or maybe the medication is wrong for you and you are even more "hyper" than you were before, feeling anxious, nervous, and upset. These may be problems that will subside with time, or they may not.

You need to talk with your physician about possible

side effects before you begin taking a medication and then be sure that you report any effects that occur after you've launched your medication trial with a new drug. Also, keep in mind that it may take quite a while to reach the right combination of dosage and medication.

Serge Mosovich, M.D., a psychopharmacologist in New York City, says that it is not that uncommon for it to take one year of work with the doctor to arrive at the best medication treatment. So keep the faith. If you are becoming impatient about finding the appropriate medication regime, you have a lot of company.

Coming Off Medication

What if you decide you no longer need to take medication for your ADD or you just want to see how you do without it? Always consult your physician to ensure that there won't be any bad effects if you suddenly quit taking your medications.

And do remember that suddenly stopping all medications is not the same as forgetting to take a pill on any given day. A total elimination of medications can have a much more radical effect on your body.

This doesn't mean that you are "addicted" to medications in the same way that people become addicted to illegal drugs such as cocaine or heroin. What it could mean, instead, is that your body has become used to the medications and that you could experience side effects without them. If you're thinking about taking a "drug holiday" (a time frame during which you don't take your medications), then be sure that you first consult the physician who prescribed the medications so that you can be warned about potential problems. This is true for all medications and is especially true for the antidepressants, which should not be withdrawn suddenly.

Changing Medication

Medical experts say that although a medication may work very well for you now—for example, an antidepressant or even Ritalin or Dexedrine (or another stimulant)—it is possible that it will not work as effectively at a later date. So keep in mind that as a result of changing circumstances and the way the medication acts on your body, you may someday need a different dose or another medication altogether.

Building Medication into Your Life

Remembering to take medication in the afternoon is a problem for many ADD people in short-acting regimes. In fact, I was repeatedly forgetting to take mine. So I got a pillbox with a built-in timer. At 3 or 4 P.M., it goes off—while I'm with an ADD patient!

Assuming that you have accepted the idea of taking medication (which may be hard for some of you), you need to build it into your routine. For example, if you are taking an evening pill, you might put the pill bottle in some obvious place (even on your pillow). Or use some other *external* prompt—a spot where you place things, an alarm, or some obvious sign. Until you become "trained," these prompts will make your life easier.

Can You Go Without Medication?

Although most experts say that a combination of medication and therapy is the best overall treatment for ADD, there are others who believe that mild forms of ADD can be treated only with therapy and behavior modification. If that works for you, then fine! Certainly you should not take medication if you and your doctor feel you don't need it. However, it has been my experience that if a person is doing without medication, the behavioral program requires a fair amount of work and may take a long time.

Support Groups, Conferences, the Internet, and Medication

Some of you may not have access to a well-run support group. Our support group in New York City is so sophisticated that we learn about groundbreaking research *before* it's published. But this knowledge can also be obtained by attending conferences—there are several adult ADD conferences each year—and by participating in Internet, or computer on-line forums. Many of these Internet sites are listed in Appendix E.

Conclusion

If you have ADD, and learning about the disorder and struggling to change your thoughts and behavior just isn't working, you may need a medication to give you that extra push. Physicians who prescribe medications for ADD often start with their own favorites, and you may find that the first medication you try helps a little, a lot, or not at all. It's possible that you may need to try several medications before you find one that works for you.

It is also true that new medications are being developed all the time. If medications available now don't help you, the medication that will help may be available in the near future.

Don't expect miracles from your medication. Even though it may help you think more clearly, be less distractible, and focus better, your symptoms will not in most cases be eradicated. In other words, you are probably going to be better, but you will still need to learn new patterns of thinking and behaving in order to bring your life to the place you want it to be.

If it works, medication can take you from wandering around in the woods to putting you on the right track. It can give you enough clarity of consciousness to address issues that you could not master. In fact, things might even be somewhat harder for you for a while. But it also may be possible to eventually achieve what you want.

7

Treating ADD with Psychotherapy, Support Groups, and Coaching

Once you've been diagnosed with ADD, it is a good idea to identify a therapist with whom you can work. Many times adults with ADD have become so mired in negative feelings about themselves that the first thing they need to do is to face these feelings directly and learn how to let them go. Besides dealing with the ADD symptoms themselves, there may be depression, anxiety, or other problems that need to be addressed.

A good therapist can also help you develop practical ways to deal with your daily life based on your own problems and circumstances. You will also develop insights into how your ADD symptoms have interacted throughout your life, which is likely to help you understand why your life has taken a certain direction. And it is our position that a good therapist will educate you thoroughly about ADD.

Experience Counts

This leads to an important issue, which I want to underscore: The ADD patient should go to a therapist with at least several years' experience in treating ADD. I say this because ADD can resemble so many other psychological diagnoses. In discussing ADD in depth with many therapist colleagues, I have discovered that most of them don't believe that ADD is a valid diagnosis with its own special issues. Some of these colleagues are senior psychotherapists with decades of experience in the field. Yet they have no real "feel" for the disorder and dismiss the issue by saying, "Oh, we are all ADD." Such a therapist cannot really be of great help to a person with ADD. Unfortunately some therapists will take on patients who believe that they have ADD—and treat them for other problems.

Learn the Therapist's Orientation

Unless the therapist is especially attuned to ADD, she will tend to fall back on whatever theory of psychotherapy she subscribes to. The therapist will search within that particular framework for a formulation and treatment plan to resolve your problems. Thus, if a therapist's favorite form of therapy is insight-oriented, he will seek to help you gain insights into the cause of your problems. Unfortunately, he will probably neglect the fact that the adult with ADD often needs to learn some concrete coping skills.

If the therapist believes primarily in cognitive therapy, then she will try to teach you how to change your thinking about yourself. Cognitive therapists will rarely seek to provide basic information on how to use an appointment book, how to manage your time, or give you rudimentary knowledge about the social cues other people send out—and which people with ADD often miss.

Unless the cognitive therapist carefully takes your ADD into consideration, you may learn to think more positively but still find yourself repeating the same mistakes because you haven't unlearned behavior that doesn't work, nor have you replaced it with behavior that does work.

Even a therapist who concentrates very heavily on changing behavior may not be aware of the extent of the ADD person's limitations and thus may assume that his suggestions will be easy for you to implement: For example, start using a (complicated) appointment book; be on time for your appointments; keep a (complicated) weekly record of your progress in dealing with a variety of issues. Anyone who knows this kind of patient would understand that such changes are not easy for a person with ADD to make. Which is another reason why your therapist, whatever their orientation, must truly understand ADD.

A major problem is that people with attention deficit disorder may have failed to learn these concrete skills in the past because, for example, they didn't have the ability to pay attention long enough to keep their appointments on time.

Or they may not have had sufficient persistence to sit down and, for example, keep a daily appointment book. In addition, the person with ADD may not have paid enough attention to the small social cues needed to make and keep friends and thus may frequently appear "out of it" in social situations; or she may be unaware of the progressive steps involved in creating and maintaining relationships.

Many therapists, however, believe that teaching such

basic skills infantilizes the adult patient and as a result they do not provide such training. However, in my ten years of working with patients with ADD, I have found the very concrete approach to be extremely effective. In fact, I would say that many of my ADD patients *need* this concrete skill training.

Also keep in mind that many therapists still practice psychoanalytic therapy, developed by Sigmund Freud during the early years of this century. Proponents of this form of therapy work with their patients to develop insights into the causes of their problems, often by linking current events to those that occurred in childhood. But for the person with ADD, it is misleading to think that the solution to his or her problems lies in an in-depth understanding of the link between childhood experiences and current problems.

Even Freud himself acknowledged the biological basis for illness, although some of his modern-day followers seem to have forgotten that. And ADD is a (neuro)biological problem.

The point here is not to consider the teaching of concrete coping skills as trivial. Building concrete skills, such as showing up for appointments, getting up on time, letting the other person know that you are really listening, finishing small tasks as a prelude to completing larger tasks—these are all necessary to building a successful life.

The Therapist with ADD

This may seem odd, but it may be valuable if the *therapist* has ADD, even though he or she may exhibit some of the same behavior as the patient—being late, having a cluttered office, forgetting appointments. (One hopes, however, that the therapist is a few steps ahead of the patient!)

Why would it be an advantage for your therapist to have ADD? When the therapist has ADD *and* is an experienced clinician, he or she can better recognize and acknowledge that ADD is a real problem for you. There is no question about whether or not the therapist takes the ADD diagnosis seriously.

Some adults with ADD may also wish to have the help of a "coach" in resolving ADD problems—for example, in reviewing goals and what has been done to achieve them. This chapter will give you information about the coaching process as well.

Diet as a Part of Treatment

Some mental health professionals believe that changing one's diet can have a positive impact on individuals with ADD—for example, eliminating or cutting back on all chemical additives in food and all processed or naturally occurring sugars. Although most professionals do not believe that ingested foods can *cause* ADD, many believe that certain foods may exacerbate the problem in a person who already has the condition.

One of my colleagues here in New York City, Richard Carlton, M.D., routinely asks his ADD patients to eliminate certain foods from their diets—chocolate, caffeine, foods containing sugar (especially sweets and desserts), and alcohol. He also recommends vitamin supplements. Dr. Carlton claims success with this treatment. I know, because I have referred several patients to him, and these diet changes can help.

Even if sugar-laden foods and other substances don't make the ADD worse, they may cause headaches and depression, which may make it appear to be more of a problem.

Finding a Good Therapist

After your physician has ruled out other medical conditions that might mimic ADD, you need to locate a good therapist as well as a psychiatrist or other medical doctor who can prescribe medication for you. Often psychologists and psychiatrists have ongoing relationships. I work with several psychopharmacologists in my area, New York City.

It's best to select your psychologist first, because this is the expert who can offer psychological testing and other screening devices. Although psychological testing is not absolutely necessary to diagnose ADD, it can provide useful information about your cognitive abilities and can also identify learning disabilities that often coexist with ADD.

One way to locate a good mental health professional is to ask support groups in your area for recommendations. For example, local chapters of the National Alliance for the Mentally Ill (NAMI) often know a great deal about local therapists and physicians. Although attention deficit disorder is not a mental illness in the usual sense of the term, it is a mild neurobiological disorder—the reason that NAMI is interested in ADD. To find the chapter nearest you, call NAMI at 800-950-NAMI.

Another important organization is Children and Adults with Attention Deficit Disorder (CH.A.D.D.), a national support group. Although most chapters of this organization concentrate on ADD in children, ask your local CH.A.D.D. leader to recommend a psychologist who treats ADD in adults.

In fact, you may be fortunate enough to have an adult chapter of CH.A.D.D. (or another organization) in your local area, and that should be a good resource. In addition, those who treat children for ADD often know of professionals who also treat adults. CH.A.D.D. has 35,000 members and 600 chapters nationwide. You can call CH.A.D.D. at 800-233-4050.

You could ask the medical doctor who may have screened you if he or she can recommend a good therapist in your area. Perhaps the doctor could ask medical colleagues for their recommendations. Your primary-care physician (internist or family practitioner) may also have some recommendations. And your clergyperson may know of a mental health professional who is experienced in this area as well.

Since your medical insurance may be paying for the psychological treatment, keep in mind that you may have a restricted choice of psychologists if you have managed care, so try to determine who is on "the list" before you begin your search. But, I will warn you, very few therapists have made a specialty of treating ADD adults.

Interviewing the Psychologist

Before you make an appointment with a psychologist you are considering, ask for a few minutes of phone time for a few short questions. Many psychologists will be willing to speak to you if you keep it brief (under ten minutes).

Ask questions such as these:

- *Do you think adults can have ADD?* (If the answer is no, cross this person off your list.)
- *Do you treat both men and women for ADD?* (If the psychologist has treated only men, a woman should think carefully before signing up.)
- *Have you ever heard of CH.A.D.D.?* (If the answer is no, this is a bad sign.)
- *About how long does it take to treat the average person with ADD?* (If the answer is "many years," think again. You may need only brief therapy for a year or so, but the exact length of therapy cannot be determined until treatment is started. However, if the psychologist has a bias toward long-term treatment, that will affect the answer.)
- *Do you work with or know any psychiatrists who can assist with the medication part of the treatment?* (The answer to this question should be yes; otherwise the psychologist may be opposed to medication.)
- *About how many adults with ADD have you treated in the last three years?* (If the answer is "one" or "two," you may need to seek out a more experienced clinician; however, if you live in a remote area, the psychologist may have treated only a few people with ADD or none at all. If the answer is "none," consider not seeing this person.)
- *About how many sessions does it take to determine if an adult has ADD?* (If the answer is "one," then it should be weighed in the context of how you feel about this therapist and whether you think

that he or she really has a handle on your problems. In many cases the psychologist needs at least
two or three sessions of therapy to determine if
you have ADD.)
- *How much does a session cost? How long does it
  last? Are your services covered under my health insurance?* (If the mental health professional you select is not covered by your insurance but is considered an excellent practitioner, you may find it
  worthwhile to pay the fees yourself.)

Don't be afraid to interview the psychologist and
don't be afraid to talk to several people. This is an
important part of your life, and you don't want to waste
your time and money seeing someone who is not competent or capable. Be honest and let the therapist know
if you feel that therapy must be limited by your time or
your pocketbook, or both, to a certain number of sessions.

Interviewing a Psychiatrist

It is also a good idea to ask such questions of the
psychiatrist or other medical doctor who might treat
your ADD. Be sure to ask the doctor about his or her
orientation. If the doctor is primarily a psychoanalyst—
a person who concentrates heavily or solely on long-
term insight-oriented work—he or she is probably the
wrong type of doctor for you.

You need a psychiatrist (or another medical doctor,
such as a neurologist or internist—if for some reason
you cannot see a psychiatrist) who believes that both
biology and genetics may play an important role in

your problems and who is willing to treat you with appropriate medications. Ideally you would see a psychopharmacologist, although such specialists generally practice in large cities. Keep in mind that medication can often be adjusted over the phone and that you need to be seen only once a month by the prescribing doctor.

Other Techniques for Evaluating Therapists

One technique recommended by some therapists is to write a letter, which includes a variety of questions, to those therapists whom you are considering. For example:

- How many adult ADD patients have you seen in the past three to five years?
- Do you work closely with a medical doctor?
- What is your orientation in psychotherapy?

In your letter be sure to explain that you are seeking some basic information that will help you select a therapist. Do *not* say that you are certain you have ADD, even if you are sure. A therapist or physician may be annoyed that a patient insists on self-diagnosing before he or she even meets you.

It's also usually a good idea to meet the therapist in person before you commit to therapy. Sometimes the therapist will be willing to see you for one session for no charge or for a reduced charge. Ask.

Types of Therapy

Different types of therapy are available to people with ADD, including individual therapy, group therapy, and support groups. For many readers, individual therapy will be the first choice.

As you explore various therapy options, there is one important principle that you should keep in mind: You must become your own advocate. Many mental health professionals really do not understand ADD, even though they may say they do. Remember: You are the consumer, and as far as I am concerned, the consumer is always right.

Many therapists are so stuck on their own pet theories that they fail to notice that their client is not getting better; and getting better is your goal. Consequently, if you try a certain therapy or therapist and it does not work for you, try an alternative. You are the boss.

Individual Therapy

Individual therapy is probably the most likely choice for the person with ADD because many people prefer the privacy of a one-to-one relationship with a mental health professional. In individual therapy you and your therapist will talk about your particular problems and develop ways in which you can deal with them more effectively.

You will probably see the psychologist once each week, although the schedule may later change. Visits usually last about forty-five to fifty minutes. After the initial screening has been completed, you and the psychologist will spend your visits talking about specific challenges, developing coping strategies, sharing new insights, and whatever concerns are on your mind.

The therapy will vary according to the psychologist's orientation. For example, the psychologist may try to help you listen to your own negative thoughts and actively challenge them. This method is central to cognitive therapy. Or the therapist may help you develop strategies for actively confronting and hopefully overcoming the ADD symptoms that have made your life less than optimal.

Often you will gain insight as the therapy proceeds. After all, you may have misunderstood your ADD and thought that you were "lazy, crazy, or stupid" (as authors Peggy Ramundo and Kate Kelly have titled their book on ADD, *You Mean I'm Not Lazy, Stupid or Crazy?!*) There may also be a number of misconceptions that have built up over the years that you can now reinterpret in the light of your new understanding of ADD.

This does not in any way release you from doing the necessary work to get your life in order. Yes, you will develop insights. But you will also need to work hard at developing skills you have never gained before.

Acknowledging Small Steps Through Therapy

Another value of seeing the therapist on an individual basis is that a good therapist can teach the ADD adult how to acknowledge the importance of small steps in making progress. Very often, people don't continue along the road of self-improvement because they don't acknowledge their small steps of progress. Instead, the person with ADD often expects a difficult problem to be solved rapidly. If it can't be solved soon, the person gives up.

This is somewhat like expecting a 250-pound woman to lose 50 pounds in a week. It can't happen. But if the obese woman were to have steady weight losses, she could eventually lose those 50 pounds. Similarly, the adult with ADD who learns the value of taking small but positive steps toward a goal learns a very valuable lesson.

The good therapist helps to keep you on track and to maintain the positive perspective needed to pursue your personal goals and improve your life.

Group Therapy

Some people may wish to supplement individual therapy with group therapy. You may gain fresh insights and new practical tips by communicating with other people who face similar problems. Group therapy is conducted by a professional therapist who leads the group and provides helpful insights into your behavior in the group. But some people don't enjoy group therapy, either because they are too shy to speak up in a group or because they don't wish to become involved in others' problems.

If group therapy is available in your area, I recommend that you consider it. But in most areas there are few groups available for ADD adults. Even here in New York City I know of only two professionals besides myself who run adult ADD groups.

My Group Therapy Sessions

I use a two-part model for group therapy. The group meets every week for an hour and a half, and over time a bond develops among the members. Professionals call this group cohesion. This group cohesion eventually becomes a healing force, and everyone in the group partakes of this mysterious energy, which helps the members devise and try out strategies to improve their own lives.

But what is special about this group (compared with other forms of group therapy) is that the first half of each session is devoted to developing concrete coping techniques and providing tips that will help members with specific ADD problems. Such techniques might include how to use an appointment book, deal with clutter in the home or office, or get up on time in the morning.

At first these strategies are taught by me. But as group cohesion develops, the members actively help each other. I am still responsible for guiding the overall process, however, since well-meaning "helpers" can sometimes become overbearing.

The other extremely valuable aspect of these groups, emphasized in the second half of the session, takes place when members communicate their concerns, worries, and vulnerabilities.

Feedback is provided in a supportive manner to encourage and empower members to work on and improve problem areas. This is immensely valuable for adults with ADD, because so many have not developed good social skills or learned the subtle social cues necessary for forming good relationships.

For example, not paying attention to a lover can ruin

the relationship. Not knowing when it is best to end a certain conversation can have disastrous effects on the job. Such small social cues are pointed out to members and taught through concrete homework assignments.

I have one warning about group therapy: ADD adults may have built up a lot of anger about how they have been treated over the years, which will come out in the group. In any group there are underlying dynamics that are sometimes not even apparent to the therapist.

For example, I was once called in to run a group of adult learning-disabled students at a local university. I (foolishly) asked them to fill out some forms at an early session. As the group progressed, an undercurrent of anger grew so strong that the group eventually broke up.

I believe that the key problem stemmed from the forms I asked them to fill out. These people had *trouble* with forms, as some people with learning disabilities do. Their anger at being asked to do something that they found so difficult was very strong; yet at the time, they were afraid to say they had trouble filling out the forms or to ask for help.

This frustration was just another enactment of many scenarios in their lives in which they were misunderstood and asked to do something they could not do. They have often been told that they were lazy or crazy for missing deadlines, or that they were stupid because they could not do something that seemed so simple.

So when these feelings are fully expressed—watch out! The level of anger, frustration, and negative feelings, and the hurt and shame, may be quite substantial. Running such a group is not for the timid!

Support Groups

Although there are nowhere near the number of support groups for ADD adults the need indicates, groups are springing up all over the country. Support groups are composed of individuals like you, and they are not usually led by a mental health professional—although some may be. In addition, they are usually very inexpensive to join and are often free. The downside of adult ADD support groups is that they may be difficult to manage, and some members may monopolize the group. The situation can become disorganized and even chaotic because it may be very difficult for leaders who have ADD to maintain order in a group whose members are all distractible.

A primary drawback to a support group is that it cannot satisfy the need for individual or group therapy. In group therapy a trained therapist guides the way and maintains perspective, especially with regard to sensitive issues, providing balance in the interactions between group members. The professional may also protect the vulnerable patient from attack or unwitting harm by other members. This guidance and protection is rarely present in support groups.

A plus in attending ADD support groups is that it can be very satisfying to learn that other people also struggle with this disorder, thus validating feelings you may have endured in isolation. You can also learn who are the best mental health professionals in your area. But keep in mind that a clinician who works well with one person may not be effective with another.

Generally speaking, support groups are safe environments, so don't be afraid to attend one. In some large cities you may find more than one such group. They may provide valuable sources of information and may also give you emotional support you've never experienced before.

Appendix D provides a listing of support groups throughout the country.

The Support Group I Attend

I have attended a sophisticated support group here in New York City for several years. Can you imagine a group of forty adult ADD people having a meeting in which they interrupt each other frequently, tap their feet, get up and walk around, ask questions off the topic, and even interrupt themselves? It is quite an experience.

But attending support groups has also taught me a great deal about the different varieties of people with adult ADD. There are quiet, thoughtful people, and there are people who are visibly restless. There are people who appear disheveled, and there are well-dressed businesspeople. There are also people who express bizarre ideas and have undergone multiple hospitalizations.

They are attorneys, high-level professionals, well-educated people and poorly educated people—all kinds of people.

These groups have also taught me how much adults with ADD have struggled. After all, it's only been in the last ten years that adult ADD has become well known or even accepted by the health care system. These people have worked very hard to seek out support systems and find solutions to their problems. If you have recently discovered that you may have ADD, you can thank the "pioneers" who have paved the way in making support groups available.

There is also valuable sharing of information about ADD. We are lucky in New York City: The group's leader is Paul Jaffe, probably one of the most knowledgeable people in the country about adult ADD, and founder of *ADDendum,* an excellent newsletter on adult ADD. So the ADD adults who attend this group are very well informed.

Education as Therapy

An important part of helping yourself as an adult with ADD is to *learn* about it. You've made a first step by reading this book, but it's a good idea to continue to learn. Ordinarily education about a disorder is not a part of therapy, but with adult ADD, it's important. By educating yourself you can learn to understand your condition more deeply, and you can be more creative in solving your problems.

Your therapist should help you learn about ADD. But it's also a good idea to find information on your own—in books and magazine articles, and from others who are knowledgeable about the topic. Be aware that professionals disagree on what are the most effective treatments or medications, so try not to overgeneralize: for example, that Ritalin is the *only* medication that works; or that unless you're in group therapy, you won't make progress. Each person is different and has a unique set of needs.

Education is also important, because once you have an understanding of ADD, you can explain it to others. They may not believe you and may even think that

ADD is an excuse for goofing off. (And let's face it, some people do use their ADD to justify their lack of behavior change.) Talk to such people about brain studies, biochemical studies, and the scientific aspects of ADD. Most people are impressed to learn that there are valid physiological differences between those people who have ADD and those who do not.

Practical Goals

To find out if you are making progress in therapy, and to focus your energies as well as the therapist's, it is helpful to identify practical and achievable goals. The next step is to develop a plan to get *there* from here. For example, most people with ADD need to bring structure into their lives. Creating structure could be accomplished by something as simple as deciding where to put your keys. Maybe you always lose them because you don't know where you put them last.

A more practical solution would be always to put the keys in the same place—your pocket or a compartment of your bag. You decide where to place them and stick to it. Let's say that you have now decided where your keys are going to "live" or call "home." (Right *there* on the dresser.) I call this an *anchor point.*

I help many of my patients develop anchor points (see also Chapter 8). This means that some aspect of their lives has an *anchor,* such as getting up at a certain time, putting their wallet or bag in a certain place so that it is always either there or with them and no place else. Creating anchor points can give you control over one or more aspects of your life, and it can enable you to move on and make even more difficult changes.

Anchor points can be aspects of time, places for things, or certain routines. For example, each morning I go through certain exercises. They warm up my body, help my lower-back problem, and make me more fit. If I don't do this routine on any given morning, I feel incomplete.

What's important to note here is that when I started this routine, I didn't want to do it. It took me a year and a half before it became a part of my life. And now that it is, I am grateful. I explain this to my adult patients with ADD: If you start to build certain *anchor points* or habits into your life, you will be more organized and able to concentrate on more important concerns.

Start with simple things. Nothing is too small, because you are giving your unconscious the message that you are controlling your life. As you move into broader issues, such as getting along with others, learning how to allow personal intimacy into your life, and other major goals, break down each challenge into specific, concrete steps. This is where the therapist can help—by laying out the sequence of steps and letting you know whether a step may be too big or too small.

Your progress in working through this step-by-step method may appear slow; and you may fail at times. No self-blame! You have had enough of that. Instead learn, build what you learn into your life—and forgive yourself if you stumble.

ADD Coaches

A new way of helping people with ADD is through *coaching*. A coach could be a mental health professional or someone in your support group or a friend or family member—although most experts believe that a family member carries too much "emotional baggage" to maintain an effective coaching relationship.

The coaching relationship is not considered a therapeutic relationship, but it deals with practical issues faced by an adult with ADD, such as organization, managing time, or goal setting. Some people use the coaching relationship in a way that is similar to my use of anchor points for the person with ADD. That is, the coaching sessions are meant to encourage the client to develop routines that will facilitate the achievement of goals.

According to Susan Sussman, codirector of the National Coaching Network, based in Lafayette, Pennsylvania, coaching can be performed in person, over the phone, or by electronic mail. Her organization has about ninety members, or "coaches," nationwide, and she can link up people with coaches in over twenty-five states. Many of her own clients live in different states, and the coaching is done by phone.

"Coaching is a one-on-one intervention that deals with practical matters around issues like time management, organizational skills, and whatever is specific to the individual," Sussman explains. "The client and the coach work together to design an alliance by looking at goals the client wants to achieve." Some clients work well with coaches who are very strong and provide numerous suggestions, she observes, while other people much prefer a quiet person who mostly listens and then offers ideas.

How long does the coaching last? It's up to you and your coach, but Sussman says that, on average, coaching lasts about six months. This varies considerably. For example, according to Sussman, one client may need coaching during the process of achieving some large goal—for example, writing a doctoral dissertation—after which the relationship would end. Another person may need something like the kind of coaching that an athlete receives, which would last throughout a professional career.

In the system discussed here, a coach generally sees the client once a week for an hour; or, if it is a telephone relationship, the coaching may occur for ten to fifteen minutes on the phone daily from Monday through Friday. Electronic mail correspondence would depend on the mutual agreement between coach and client, but it would take place at least weekly.

Another coaching system is LifeCoach, founded by Edward Hallowell, M.D., the senior author of *Driven to Distraction,* an excellent book about adult ADD. He has overseen the development of the organization, which is headed by Josselyn Bliss, a therapist and mother of two ADD children. One advantage of this coaching system is that it was specifically designed for ADD adults.

This system is structured as follows: Client and coach have an initial hour-long session over the phone to assess the issues on which the client wants to focus and to obtain background information. Then a coach is assigned, and a time is scheduled for the client's daily call to the coach to review goals and progress. The client signs up for two weeks at a time and renews by credit card.

I have participated in this system myself, and it seems well designed. For example, if the client forgets to call, the coach will call the client collect—a disincentive—five minutes after the call should have been made. Clients are also asked to sign a contract, and it is made very clear to them that coaching is not psycho-therapy.

Another coaching system is available as an electronic pager. Called NeuroPage, it is a small pager worn by the client that can sound an alarm, vibrate on a person's belt, or do both. The client also has the option of not having an alarm go off that might disturb others.

A message shows up on the pager's small electronic screen for about forty seconds. Any message can be programmed into the computer system, which will page the client daily, with up to twelve messages a day. Costs vary with the contract, but the schedule I've discussed with the East Coast director costs $105 a month; the start-up cost is $200. This system is especially useful for people with significant memory problems.

I am not aware of any research that has evaluated the effectiveness of these coaching systems. But they seem to be an excellent way of adapting to the needs of the ADD adult. That is, ADD adults typically need *daily* prodding and support to maintain a focus on their goals. The traditional system of once-a-week therapy may involve a much longer process with ADD adults than a daily system such as coaching.

Controversial Treatments

A variety of treatments have gained media attention, but they have not been researched sufficiently to determine their overall effectiveness. Here are a few.

Nonpharmacological Treatments

Some people have insisted that nonpharmaceutical treatments, such as vigorous exercise or changing one's diet, can help resolve ADD. Some people believe that certain foods or substances such as sugar can actually cause ADD in a child or an adult. It's possible that this could be true in a small percentage of cases, but studies have shown that for most people dietary changes alone do not lead to large improvements with ADD.

This needs some qualification, however. Years ago the Feingold diet was a popular method for relieving symptoms in children with ADD, and it has attracted a following of professionals and parents. They swear by the Feingold principles, which include eliminating food additives as well as certain foods that they believe may cause allergies in some people.

Richard Carlton, M.D., a psychopharmacologist in New York City, begins his treatment of ADD adults by having them eliminate certain foods, including chocolate—a substance to which some people with ADD are very sensitive—and any foods that contain salicylates, such as apples. Sometimes these patients can have very good results. According to my understanding, however, research has not shown the Feingold diet to be particularly effective for a large number of people with ADD.

Exercising Your ADD Away?

Exercise, although advisable for most adults, can only provide temporary (if any) relief from ADD symptoms, and most people will need medication as well. It should be noted, however, that if you experience anxiety or depression along with ADD, exercise can be beneficial.

Exercise may serve an additional purpose: It helps to burn up excessive energy and can actually serve as a form of self-medication. How? Vigorous exercise can biochemically stimulate the body to create internal chemicals called endorphins, giving the person a natural high. Medical experts advise that exercise can even help people who are mildly depressed. Some experts who treat ADD adults, such as Ed Hallowell, strongly recommend that they establish a regular exercise routine, for all of the above reasons.

For the ADD adult who has insomnia, exercising before bedtime may relax the person sufficiently so that he can drift off to sleep without medication.

"Natural" Preparations

There are some vitamins or herbal preparations that may promise a natural "cure" for ADD. Please be very careful with such preparations. Because of current laws the Federal Drug Administration (FDA) does not regulate herbal or homeopathic preparations, and the quality and contents of a drug sold in a health food store may be questionable. At present, I am not aware of studies indicating that "natural" vitamins or herbal preparations will work for ADD adults. It's possible that they *may* work, but we don't know at this time. Nor do we know the long-term effects of taking such substances.

EEG Biofeedback

Some proponents believe that children can be trained to increase or alter their brain waves and thus affect their ADD. Studies have involved only small numbers of children and no control groups, so there isn't enough supporting evidence to recommend this therapy.

The major proponent of the neurofeedback method is Joel Lubar, Ph.D., who runs a biofeedback clinic in Tennessee. Although he has published papers on using the technology with ADD people, his research methods have been criticized on several points by Dr. Russell Barkley, an eminent researcher in the field (see Barkley's April 1992 article). An interesting personal account by Paul Jaffe can be found in *ADDendum* 9.

Applied Kinesiology

Also called the neural organization method, applied kinesiology is a chiropractic procedure performed on the skull. It is based on the theory that ADD is caused by a misalignment and that if the misalignment is adjusted by a chiropractor, the problem will go away. I am aware of no scientific evidence to support this theory, and I caution the consumer.

Conclusion

There are a number of treatment strategies for adults with ADD. The most well known are medication and psychotherapy. Medication, of course, has to be prescribed by a medical doctor (usually a psychiatrist), and psychotherapy can be done with a psychiatrist, psychologist, or other therapist. The important issue in psychotherapy is to select someone who has substantial experience in treating adult ADD patients. Group therapy can be useful if it takes into account the special needs of the person with ADD. Support groups can also be useful, especially for emotional support, information about the leading professionals in your area, and education about ADD. Coaching is useful for some people, and focuses on resolving more concrete issues than those that are treated in psychotherapy. For some people, changing and purifying the diet can be effective. Other treatments, such as EEG biofeedback training, herbal preparations, and chiropractic, have been put forth, although scientific evidence has not yet been found to support their efficacy.

8

Tips, Techniques, and Strategies for Overcoming ADD

We have just reviewed some of the basic elements of treatment—medication, psychotherapy, support groups, and coaching. To give you a framework for the "whole package," I borrow from Ed Hallowell and John Ratey's overview of the components of treatment for ADD adults:

- Medication
- Supportive therapy, including education and support groups
- Structured behavioral management, including coaching
- Cognitive remediation
- Group therapy
- Involvement of couples or significant others in therapy

Even though you may be on a very effective medication regime for your ADD and you see a helpful therapist on a regular basis, you will probably need to incorporate some coping mechanisms, tips, and techniques into your everyday life. These can include the use of physical reminders and tools, principles and techniques of time management, and some concrete interpersonal skills that you can practice. These pointers can be examined under the general category of "Structure."

This chapter discusses the components of structure as well as some of the basic tools—both nonelectronic and high-tech—that can help people with ADD incorporate structure into their lives.

The Importance of Structure

One characteristic of ADD adults is that their ability to pay attention is not as strong as their other abilities. In many cases, their attention may be spotty or inconsistent. Adults with the impulsive type of ADD may not think before acting or speaking. Then it's too late; the embarrassment is there for all the world to see. Creating structure—the means of organizing or shaping our tasks and lives—is a way to keep attention and behavior within certain serviceable boundaries.

There have always been a variety of structures in place to help a person give order and meaning to the different phases of life. These have included ceremonies for getting married or becoming a "man" (such as the bar mitzvah) or various other coming-of-age rituals. Today there are structures that enable us to manage time, such as regular school or work hours, the typical nine-to-five work day. Our progress through high school college and beyond is marked by certain external structures (examinations, graduation, diploma or degree, the dissertation) as is training in certain professions, which culminates in a license.

Many of us may not have appreciated some of these

structures, and we may even have considered giving up a goal because the path to its achievement seemed too rocky. But many times we persisted and did what we had to do because we benefited from the very structures and rules of the system. Looking back, we might be glad we stayed in the game and completed what was necessary. However, many ADD people cannot sustain their efforts and attention over time and thus do not reach their goals.

One problem today is that many helpful structures that were in place for years have eroded, and people now have to rely far more on creating their own ways of shaping and organizing their activities and projects. As a result, if we are smart ADD people, we will consciously and willingly bring structure back into our lives.

Structure is extremely valuable to the adult with ADD. It helps us to avoid chaos. We know, for example, that children who are ADD or learning disabled can benefit greatly from highly structured environments. The same can be true for ADD adults.

If you acknowledge the validity of this concept, you can then become creative in devising solutions to your own problems. Much of the literature on adult ADD states that people with ADD can be more creative than the average person. Here's your chance! (And be sure to tell me about your success stories.)

We can look at the concept of structure in terms of putting boundaries around something, in the way we put up walls in a building to keep out the cold and to give people a place to carry out their daily activities. An example of an item used to create structure is the timer, which places a time limit on a certain activity. In the same way, a deadline uses a date to place a boundary on an activity or a project. If you set up these boundaries or structures, they may enhance your ability to achieve your goals. They may help to *contain* your attention so that you can do what you want to do.

Tips on Building Structure into Your Life

As you start to create structure to control the chaos in your life, look at these tools as neutral, even helpful, objects. For example, being on time, using an appointment book, or using a timer to limit certain activities are not "uncool." They are simply tools to help you achieve your goals. If it takes six alarm clocks to get you up in the morning, then *use six alarm clocks*. Maybe you can eventually reduce this small army to four alarm clocks, then two, and finally just one big, loud alarm clock that you can hear across a room! You are not defective because you need such tools to structure your life. They are helping you to be more effective in achieving your goals.

Other external devices are calendars or hand-carried organizers or whiteboards (also called dry-erase boards). Or you may opt for a variety of innovative computer solutions, such as software to help you organize your time or the new electronic organizers. For example, Timex has a programmable watch to remind you to take your medication, go to that appointment, and so forth. It also stores phone numbers and to-do lists.

The Evening Assessment

One technique that I have suggested to several of my patients during the last few years is what I call the evening assessment. This refers to a period of time at the end of the day in which you collect your thoughts on how the day has gone, what you did well, what you might have done better—and what you might have forgotten altogether. Be sure to be positive and to compliment yourself, especially if you are working on a new skill, developing some new behavior, or facing an issue that you have avoided before.

The period of time for the evening assessment should be long enough to actually get several thoughts together, but not so long as to make it laborious. People differ in how they use this time, and each day requires its own specific time period that is just right. But I say not less than five minutes, and not longer than thirty.

For those people who are able to keep a journal, it is a terrific way to keep track of your progress. Writing down your evaluation of the day will make it sharp and real. I realize that many ADD people have illegible handwriting (which often improves after medication), or they may otherwise not be inclined to keep a journal. If this is true for you, give it a try, even if your journal entries are only occasional: It could become a valuable tool.

The evening assessment may also be used to plan for the next day. One technique that many counselors suggest in order to have a more peaceful sleep is to write down the things that you are going to do tomorrow. In fact, write down six things. This makes for more restful sleep for some people: They will not be tossing and turning over what they have to do the next day.

Organizational Tools

Lists

Many people with ADD swear by lists that they make as well as little messages on Post-It notes that they write to themselves. One man says that he writes his lists and messages on whiteboards scattered about his home and office. Once he wrote himself a note on the bathroom mirror! Lists are an important and common structure or device that can be effective in helping the ADD person develop control over his or her activities and time.

This method, like the others presented in this chapter, needs to be worked on over time in order to become an effective tool. Don't expect overnight success. Often there is a training period, like the time when you had training wheels on your first bike or when you learned how to play tennis: Practice, practice, practice.

You might also be able to get some help from a fellow support-group member. Arrange to call each other to see how you are both managing the lists, organizers, or other means of creating structure in your life. Besides, having another person involved in your growth can be a fun way to work on self-improvement. Be sure to stick to business, however.

Calendars and Appointment Books

In our hectic world today, we may have many pressing professional and personal commitments, and some of us may be booked months ahead. Few of us, whether with or without ADD, could remember every single obligation we must meet during a period of several months. Which is why a calendar works—either a hardcopy version on which you write down your appointments or a software calendar that might be combined with other operations.

Many of my adult patients with ADD have found it very beneficial to develop the use of appointment books or the more elaborate organizers that I will describe later. You may never have worked with calendars or appointment books before; or even if you used them, you may not have developed your skills to the point where these devices truly helped you to manage your time and your life.

In my professional practice I have found that it can take a long time for the ADD person to learn to use an appointment book or calendar effectively. What you are trying to correct are long-standing habits, and your entire lifestyle may be built around some of them. For example, one freelance photographer with ADD never adjusted to the demands of a regular schedule because he never learned to manage his time well. So his only alternative was to be his own boss.

One of the biggest problems faced by ADD adults is time management. Many ADD people are often late to appointments—if they show up at all. Also, the person with ADD often estimates that tasks can be completed a lot faster than is really possible. So they overcommit to a number of projects and then squeeze their time so that all the projects suffer.

If you have trouble managing your time, create a system and keep at it—perhaps with some help. It may take you a while before you are good at your new system, and you may decide to change the system to one that works better. That is all right. Keep at it until you have something that works for you.

Notebook Organizers

Many people swear by their organizers and say that they would be lost without this book full of addresses, phone numbers, appointments, and planning sheets. A person with ADD might be daunted by some of these elaborate organizers, with sections for daily appointments, monthly calendars, yearly plans, projects, graph paper, notes, business-card holders, six categories of to-do lists, and more.

In principle such organizers could be valuable tools for adults with ADD. But the problem is that, with so many sections and tabs and different kinds of papers, such an organizer could overload the circuits of even the most ambitious person wishing to organize his or her life. In that case, you might be advised to start with one of the simpler organizers, one that doesn't immediately throw you into a panic.

Commercial organizers can be purchased at large stationery stores, and some brand names are Day-Timer, Franklin, Day Runner™, Filofax, Rolodex, and others. If such a system works for you, it can be a tremendous asset in your life.

Most ADD people who use organizers and with whom I have worked report that they need to spend about thirty minutes each day with these notebooks. They look at what they have done during the previous day and plan what they need to do for the next few days. This is all done in the context of larger goals they have created for their lives—and written down in their "Goals" section.

One young man with whom I worked, who is a successful computer professional (and learning disabled), went through six different elaborate organizer notebook systems before he settled on one that works for him. And now the other five are in the closet! But it is probably his sheer tenacity at organizing his goals that gained him a coveted job as head of computer networking for a multibillion-dollar corporation (and without a college degree, I might add). He spends about thirty minutes each day planning his activities, and this exercise has made him very effective in organizing them with respect to carefully formulated, written goals.

Ideally, the organizer is a system that has as its focus large-scale goals, which in turn are broken down into systematic actions so that day-to-day activities relate directly to the broader, visionary goals.

The larger goals may be so substantial that they might seem beyond reach if simply written on paper: creating an institute, finding the ideal mate, starting a business, developing a career, or writing a book. By using an organizer effectively you can break down your big dreams into day-to-day activities and eventually realize them.

Don't kid yourself! This takes time and effort. It may take a year before your organizer works effectively for you. Considering that you might succeed in making your day-to-day activities align with what you truly want in life, all the effort will be worth it.

Support Groups

Before reading this book, you may not have been aware that there are hundreds of support groups nationwide for people with ADD and for parents who have children with ADD. Such a group could be invaluable for you. Finally, you can meet others who really understand your problem and who not only acknowledge the problem but have had experiences similar to yours. It can be a great relief not only to swap stories with like-minded people but also to learn what solutions have worked for them that you can try. We have compiled an extensive list of adult ADD groups in Appendix D.

We explored the difference between support and therapy groups in Chapter 7. Both groups can be thought of as external structures that may be a source of information, inspiration, friends, tips, and recommendations of the best doctors and therapists in the area.

You may also use such a group to find a partner to check on your mutual list making, time management, use of organizers, and other behaviors you want to improve. This may not work for a variety of reasons—personality conflicts, forgetting to call each other, one person pushing unwanted advice on the other, and the like. But many times it can work.

Again, one of the themes of this book is that you should never give up. If one strategy doesn't work after you've really given it a try, then try another—and another. But give each one a good shot.

Confronting Your Clutter: Using Professional Organizers

Some adults with ADD may want to hire a person who is an expert at organizing other people's homes and offices. In fact, there is an association of organizers from whom you can get the names of people in your area. Yes, there are people who are professional organizers!

The way they work is to come to your home or office and help you find a place for everything. Besides this cleanup phase, the organizer usually helps you develop systems for maintaining your surroundings in an organized state. In hiring the organizer you need to be willing to commit to following the system that you and the organizer create for your environment. It needs to be easily understood and adapted to your own particular needs. All of this sounds very logical. But if you are a disorganized person, it may take more effort than you imagine.

Before hiring a professional organizer, you should interview the person directly and find out how he or she works. Explain that you have ADD, that you have a problem with organization and need a system that is not complicated and is easy to follow. In addition, don't hire anyone who treats you like a recalcitrant child. You're simply an adult with an organization problem. After all, you're smart enough to hire someone to help you.

I have worked with about eight different personal organizers, and all were effective in some way. But there are some ways you can maximize your progress. The first thing you need to do is to be clear about why you need an organizer. You may know how to file things but you can't seem to manage the time to do the filing. Or you may really not have a good sense of where things belong.

You may have trouble categorizing papers according to specific topics or figuring out what order to put them in. Or you may just need someone to help you focus because, when it comes right down to it, you know how to do everything but you just don't do it. Once you have defined the problem, you can find the organizer who's best for you.

I have found that most organizers are willing to discuss your needs over the phone. You can break down the particular type of organizing you require into categories such as closets, billing, financial, space and interiors, or time management.

The next consideration is price. I have found that, as of this writing, most organizers in the New York area charge about $40 an hour. Some people who specialize in organizing businesses may charge $50 to $100 per hour.

Also keep in mind that working with your organizer is a time-intensive process. If you must go through most of your belongings and if, like most people with ADD, you have *big-time trouble* with clutter, then you have twenty to one hundred hours ahead of you until you get organized.

Keep in mind that no one but you can go through your stuff and put it where you want it to be. You may have to consult with your organizer about finding the right place for things, but eventually you have to decide where everything should go.

Surprisingly many professional organizers are unaware of adult ADD. And yet adults with ADD represent a rich marketplace for professional organizers! I attended an adult ADD conference several years ago, and one of the most packed workshops—several hundred people and standing-room only—was the one dealing with clutter.

Maybe you can make a deal with your professional organizer: For every new client you bring in that pays him or her for five hours, you get an hour free. You could also give her a copy of this book or other books recommended in the appendix. As the organizer becomes more knowledgeable about ADD, he will be better able to help you and others with ADD.

Get a Clutter Buddy

Another option is to trade time with another person who also wants to work on reducing clutter. I recently made a deal with a neighbor that if she would sit quietly on my couch for two hours and do something (like paying her bills or writing letters), I would do the same for her. So there she sat—quietly—for two hours. Then the timer went off, and we both got up and went to her apartment, where I sat quietly for two hours and she organized. That's all we needed—another person there to keep us focused. It cost us nothing but time. Actually we were both doing productive activities in both apartments. This brings up an important issue for some, perhaps most, ADD people: They know what to do, but they don't do it. By having another person in the room with them—even sitting quietly—they are more motivated to complete organizational tasks.

To find a professional organizer in your area, contact the National Association of Professional Organizers, a nationwide organization with about seven hundred members.

The Action Board

David Viscott, M.D., a well-known TV psychiatrist in Los Angeles, has a wonderful way of organizing projects that might also be useful to the ADD adult. Get a large bulletin board and a lot of bright, colored cards (3×5, or 4×6; now in neon colors). Put your tasks on the colored cards, one task per card, and arrange the cards in a separate vertical column for each project. So you have several columns of cards, each column a different color. As you finish one task, remove the card from the board, and move up the other cards. Put the new task card below the ones that have higher priority. Some people put pictures of things that they want on the Action Board—for example, a picture of their ideal house.

This method takes advantage of the idea of using an external, visible structure to help you organize your activities or plans in a rational way. The bright colors will also catch your eye and focus your attention on the things you need to do in your life—and in the order you need to get them done. Be sure to put the board in a place where you will notice it!

Electronic Solutions

White-Noise Generators

Often people with ADD may be very distracted by noise in the work environment that others automatically tune out. One possible solution could be a white-noise generator, which can mask the sounds that prevent the ADDer from concentrating. It need not be a costly device—a plain electric fan will often suffice to do the job. Or an air purifier could purify your office air as well as serve as a white-noise generator.

In some cases, people with ADD have great difficulty both getting to sleep and waking up in the morning. One possible solution to the problem with falling asleep could be the white-noise generator, which can help screen out external noise and allow the person to relax.

It is possible, however, that much of the problem in falling asleep is internal to the person rather than caused by the external environment. In such cases the person with ADD may benefit from learning to relax the body progressively and allow herself to drift off to sleep.

Electronic Organizers

One solution to the problem of forgetting or losing a hard-copy organizer is a computerized organizer. There are many such organizers, and some of them are very elaborate. There are both small computers you can carry around and software programs for your PC that can help you to become more organized.

Sharp produces a whole series of organizers small enough to carry in your pocket or purse, which, as of this writing, range drastically in price from about $20 to $600. Casio and Franklin make some handheld organizers. Royal offers a Personal Organizer that includes a phone directory, scheduler, calculator, and alarm clock; and it also gives you the option of writing short memos to yourself.

One helpful thing about these devices is that they can be used to remind you to take your medication, which is a frequent problem for people with ADD. Many people with ADD enjoy computers, and the idea of using an organizer that is also a small computer may be exciting to you.

There is a downside, however. Some of these devices may be expensive, although the price could be justified if the person is greatly helped. But the other more serious problem is that people with ADD often lose things.

I once did therapy with a young ADD man who left his expensive camera on top of his car. He drove away, but remembered it an hour later. Too late. The camera was gone—and was probably in pieces. When this young man pressed his parents to buy him an expensive electronic organizer, they reminded him of this incident. He agreed that he would be better off with a paper version.

Software Programs

Despite the disadvantages, technology can be a useful tool in organizing. Software programs can help people with ADD to organize their lives. Day-Timer Technologies in San Mateo, California, released Day-Timer Organizer 2.0 in late 1995. This software offers scheduling, task management, expense tracking, an address book, and other functions.

Another advantage to adults with ADD is that once you've installed this program, you probably won't lose your personal computer; so you will have it ready when you need it. This software is priced at about $60 as of this writing.

Another organizer software is Lotus Organizer, offered by the Lotus Development Corporation. This program offers you a calendar, project manager, address book, to-do list, and many more options. This product costs about $150.

There are also many organizer or PIM programs for the Macintosh. Some of the most popular are In Control, Now Up To Date, Day Timer, and others. Check with your computer store and review the latest computer magazines to find what may work well for you.

Timex™ Datalink Watch

"I think this relationship may actually last because of this device," said one ADD man of his Timex Datalink watch in reference to his current relationship with a woman he is dating. Dating was extremely difficult for him because he'd lose phone numbers, forget what time (and sometimes where) he was supposed to pick up his date; and even though he told his dates he had ADD, they were unsympathetic.

Now, by having this special watch interface with his computer, he has successfully programmed phone numbers into his watch as well as important appointment dates and times, to-do lists, and upcoming events. He has also programmed the alarm in his watch to remind him of appointments by beeping at appropriate intervals. There could even be a wedding in the future for this man!

Using a Timer

I often can get distracted by many different things in my office and home environments. So I use a timer to structure my time and to keep on task. I set it for a time that I feel is appropriate for the task. When the beeper goes off, I then take a break, again for a specified period of time. This helps to compartmentalize my time into chunks, which I can arrange according to tasks or activities I need or want to focus on. I recently got a new gizmo. It's a pocket organizer, and I can set all kinds of alarms to remind me of things to do during the day. It actually makes the idea of timing myself fun.

Another suggestion—for managing time nonelectronically—that I offer some of my ADD patients concerns what I call *composing time,* or *composing moments.* Take a short period of time in which you try to compose yourself, to let yourself settle down. Let your thoughts become as quiet as possible. This is especially useful if you are in the midst of a frazzling situation. You can understand this as simply taking a break, as many of us do every workday. What I want to convey is that you do something deliberate and conscious to pull yourself out of a *big-time frazzle.*

On-line Computer Groups

A variety of help is available to the adult ADDer who has on-line access to computer groups. (You need a computer and a modem to connect with such groups.) For example, CompuServe, a service to which you can subscribe, has a very active ADD forum where people send and receive messages and which also includes a helpful "library" of files related to ADD. You can also access the ADD Internet newsgroup (News:alt.support.attn-deficit) through CompuServe or through the Internet.

Do keep in mind, however, that unless you use private E-mail directed to an individual, what you say on the forum or on the Internet can be read by anyone who chooses to read it. As a result, you may wish to avoid divulging too much personal information. This is also very important for the impulsive ADDer to keep in mind when leaving a message for another forum member in public.

There are also increasing numbers of "web pages" on the Internet itself for the person with ADD. (See Appendix E for a listing of several key groups.) In fact, on-line communication can be ideal for the adult with ADD—you can leave messages when you feel like it and you can later pick up responses when it is convenient for you to do so.

Be on Your Guard About Electronic Solutions

Don't be lulled into thinking that an electronic device will help resolve your ADD symptoms. I know one doctor who always recommends a particular electronic organizer for his patients. What he doesn't recognize is that even if they do use this device to remind them to take their medication, patients may (1) immediately turn it off and forget the reminder, (2) forget to carry along the device in the first place, (3) forget to program the device to beep as a reminder to take the medication, (4) forget to put the device in a place where they can hear it, or (5) drop it and break it. Once I said to this therapist, "Sometimes I wish you had ADD. Then you might understand that these problems are not solved by gizmos. They are solved by consciousness." I still don't know if he got it.

ADD is a problem with many facets—a different biochemistry, inconsistent consciousness, unwanted behaviors, problems with time management, and so on.

So if these devices don't work for you, it may not be your fault.

I have worked with computer programs for years (on the Macintosh) and have found some of them helpful. But more than half of them have been very disappointing. Computer programs are sometimes difficult to learn (unless you are a computer maven, or expert); and if they become locked up or "bomb" on you (which has happened to me), your information is inaccessible or, even worse, may be lost forever. Your electronic equipment may also not be with you all the time, so the information is not always available.

Therefore, I have recently returned to a paper-and-pencil organizer of my own design. I use standard loose-leaf stationery and simple items that can be found in any stationery store—dividers with the plastic tabs that you used in high school, and little plastic bags to hold paper clips.

I have found this loose-leaf method beneficial in the following ways:

- I can carry it with me wherever I go; computers, even laptops, are too heavy.
- Materials are cheap (about $10 for paper and other materials).
- I can drop my organizer and it won't break.
- Its standard size will accommodate articles in the notebook (especially if it has inside pockets).
- I can scribble in my notebook anytime I have a thought.

The downside is that a standard-size notebook is still fairly large; many young people and most women find it cumbersome. And it is not as fun to play with as the electronic helpers.

Besides, I've come to the conclusion that it doesn't matter what system you choose to help you organize your life. What matters is *what you do* to develop the system. The device will not do it for you. Only *you* can make it work—day after day. But you mustn't become obsessed with the system. The point is simply to work on developing a system, or systems, that will improve your life and advance your goals.

Before you choose an organizing system, do what is called a *criterion measure*. That is, if your system would work as it is intended, what would be some obvious effects on your life? And how long would it take for you to see these results? Put this down in your journal. And remind yourself to check your calendar to see whether use of your system has brought you the desired results. Let's try out this little system right here:

TODAY'S DATE	RESULTS THAT SHOW THE SYSTEM IS WORKING	DUE DATE
_____	_____	_____
_____	_____	_____

Now you have a way of checking whether or not the organizing system you have developed is working. Place a marker on this chart, and check your progress on the "due date." Is your organizing system working for you? If not, revise your strategy. *And never give up!*

Other Suggestions for People with ADD

Adults with ADD say that if you think you have ADD, don't procrastinate and keep wondering about it! Get a diagnosis. If you do have ADD, obtain the treatment you need. But don't presume that *learning* that you have ADD is the magic answer to all of your problems. You may well have to make some major changes in your life.

For example, you may have a sedentary indoor job when you would be better suited to an outdoor job that demands plenty of physical activity. Rather than being a clerk you might do better as a salesperson.

There are many practical steps you can take to improve your life when you have ADD. You will find some concrete advice in the following section.

Make Others Aware of Your ADD

A very helpful approach to coping with ADD is to make others aware of its characteristics so that they can better understand and relate to you. M. White (1994) frames the issue by having an adult with ADD directly address a friend or significant person in his or her life:

- "I may forget to complete a task, but don't take it personally."
- "I need to do things in my own way, which may not be the most usual way of doing things."
- "I may be overstimulated by certain social situations."
- "I am sometimes impulsive and may hurt your feelings unintentionally."

- "I may overcommit myself and fail to schedule my time realistically."

This list reads like a kind of confession, the ADD adult's plea for understanding from those people who are important in his or her life. Although someone who has long been around an ADD person may in fact be aware of these issues, it may still be quite a step for the adult ADDer to read this list aloud. I would not be surprised if it evokes a deep response.

Try to Work in a Clean Space

Avoid clutter whenever possible and try to maintain a "clean desk" policy. "Keep your work areas and living areas clean," Jerry advises others with ADD. He bases this view on his own life. "I have noticed that the messier my apartment is, the less motivated I am."

Avoid Television

Another man with ADD avoids television, and he advises other ADD adults to follow his example. "TV is the downfall of the ADDer," he says. "When I sit down in front of the TV, it is so easy for me to go into this mindless state. TV doesn't hold my attention. Instead I just zone out in front of it."

Finish One Project Before Starting a New One

This advice may be difficult for most people with ADD, who are easily diverted from what they're currently working on by the siren song of other exciting projects. But what often happens is that you have many different projects going all at once, and nothing gets done. I heard one anecdote of a woman complaining that her husband with ADD had torn down a wall, but hadn't yet fixed it after a week. Her friend sympathized.

"You don't understand!" she said. "It's an *outside* wall!"

Create Anchor Points

Many people with ADD lose their keys, their watches, their glasses, and other items, primarily because they put them down wherever they are at the moment. People with ADD need to unlearn this habit if it is one of the things that makes their lives chaotic. Instead, make a conscious effort to create *anchor points,* places where certain items belong and where you will always put them. (Anchor points are also discussed in Chapter 7.) For example, one anchor point could be a place you always want to keep your wallet. If you are out doing errands, keep the wallet only in one pocket or a certain part of your bag. Some people actually put up a little wall hanger labeled "Keys," and this is where they put them when they arrive home. Or you could decide always to put your glasses on your nightstand or next to your computer.

If just thinking about it doesn't do the trick, then write it down on a piece of paper. Write down the object and the place where it belongs on a small chart. If this doesn't work, you can use a behavioral-therapy method known as overcorrection.

Overcorrection

I once had a patient, Louise, who kept leaving her keys in the door; then she'd go into her house and forget the keys. She did it at least four times a week. We developed an overcorrection program and, after two weeks, she was making this mistake only once a week; two weeks later she was making this mistake only once a week. After two more weeks of overcorrection, she was making this mistake only once a month.

I had Louise open the door and then immediately place her keys in "their spot" (the anchor point). This was the only place where the keys would "live" in her house. Then she might do something nice—but brief— such as getting a hug from her husband. (He was very cooperative.) Then she would go outside again, open the door, and put the keys on the hook—over and over again.

She repeated this routine ten times a day for two weeks. Most of those times, her husband would be there to give her a hug after she put the keys in their "rightful" place. I asked Louise if she thought the program worked. She blushed a little, saying, "Well, we hardly ever got past the fourth trial." They had a good relationship, but the husband was a little *too* cooperative.

Overcorrection means practicing something so much that you pound it into your consciousness. You are trying to lay down behavioral tracks in your brain that are so durable that the actions they trace become habitual.

Driving with ADD

Unfortunately, studies have revealed that adolescents and young men with ADD are more likely to be involved in car accidents and to receive traffic tickets than their peers without ADD. So advice for ADD adults who drive is really important in any self-help book.

One study compared the driving of thirty-five people with ADD (ages sixteen to twenty-two) with that of thirty-six control subjects without ADD. (This study was published in the August 1993 issue of *Pediatrics.*) Researchers found that the people with ADD were involved in more accidents and received more injuries during those accidents than did the non-ADD group. In addition, the ADD group was more likely to have caused the accident than the non-ADD group. The ADD group also had a higher rate of speeding (and speeding citations) than did the non-ADD group.

A subgroup with an even higher rate of problem driving habits is the group of ADD teenagers who were also diagnosed with either oppositional defiant disorder or conduct disorder. (These two disorders are frequently diagnosed among children with serious behavioral problems.)

As a result, several suggestions offered in *The Med-ADD Review* might be well worth considering. Women with ADD should also read these suggestions. (Women with ADD may have a high rate of traffic accidents and citations, too; they just haven't been studied yet.)

- Try to avoid the rush-hour traffic whenever you can.

- Know where you're going. Have clear directions before you leave.
- Don't use your cell phone while driving. Pay attention to the traffic around you.
- Don't place anything on top of the car before you leave! You'll probably forget it's there and it will go flying off as you drive away. This could be very dangerous.
- Give yourself enough time to arrive at your destination.

Accommodations on the Job

Don't forget that when you have ADD, you are also covered under the Americans with Disabilities Act (ADA), which requires most employers to accommodate workers with disabilities. It might not have occurred to you, but ADD is considered a disability. However, there are several issues to consider here.

First, the employer must know that you have ADD before any accommodations can be made, and some employees are reluctant to reveal this information.

One man employed in the security field was diagnosed with ADD. He faced regular drug-screening tests as a condition of his employment and felt compelled to reveal his ADD to his employer because he knew that his ADD medication would show up in the screening. If he did not notify his employer, he would be considered a substance abuser. If you are subject to drug screenings, you can prove to your employer that you are taking a prescribed medication and thus may not risk being fired from your job.

Most of us are not subject to drug screening and thus

are not really compelled to tell the boss about our ADD. In addition, you may feel ashamed or embarrassed about the ADD and try to "tough it out," or keep the problem a secret. For example, you work overtime, trying to minimize the piles of work that ADDers are notorious for accumulating, and you may live in fear that you'll be discovered. Bad idea.

If you have ADD and you need accommodations on the job, it's a good idea to come up with a plan for workplace adaptations. For example, would you be more productive if you came in early or late or had flexible hours that gave you more time alone to concentrate? Do you become so distracted by having other people around that you need to work in a cubicle or room by yourself? Do you need frequent breaks to walk around and get rid of excessive energy?

Do you need extra time to perform some tasks? In one case a man sued, and won, for the right to have extra time to take his bar examination because he had ADD and worked at a slower pace than others. In fact, I have performed several official evaluations for learning-disabled adults to enable them to have extra time on the bar examination or entrance exams for college or graduate school. I have even helped doctors get extra time on their board exams. Yes, they, too, sometimes need accommodations.

Try to determine what your key problems are and what, if anything and within reason, the employer might be able to do to accommodate you. Keep in mind that just because you have ADD does not automatically qualify you for extensive (or any) accommodations.

Saying Hello to Reality

Sometimes when ADD adults get better, they experience a rude awakening to reality. They come out of their fantasy cloud and realize the hard truth: Much of life is hard.

I had a patient—let's call him Bob—who came to see me because he believed that his procrastination and inefficiency resulted from traumatic experiences in childhood. He had read part of a popular magazine article on eye movement desensitization reprogramming (EMDR)—in which I have been trained—and wanted my help in lifting away the alleged traumatic events.

It turned out he was a dramatic case of ADD. At forty-seven years of age, he had not gotten very far in his career, despite being an Ivy League graduate. He had ongoing fantasies of inventing some widget (although he had no idea what it could be), selling the Widget Company for several million dollars, and retiring to a beach in Florida, where he would sip his mint juleps as he watched the sun set. He had no specific plans, no particular design abilities that I could observe, and very little discipline to sit down and do what was necessary to start up a business.

After some neuropsychological testing he was started on medication. Once he had become stabilized on the medication, he came to see that he had been living in a fantasy world, which included remarkably unrealistic views about how he might make his fortune. Part of our therapy was intended not only to have him face such issues as "working hard to get what you want" but also to help him change his frame of mind so that he could *enjoy* the process of working hard and realize that he was creating something that had never existed before.

One of the indications of success in the psychotherapy of ADD adults might be their "walking" in a new and truer reality, one that they had never fully confronted in their "foggy" ADD consciousness.

The Walk of Integrity

After you have been diagnosed and begun treatment, there is a tendency for you to say to yourself and others, "Oh, there goes my ADD again." This becomes a universal excuse machine. It puts the blame on your condition, as if you were some kind of victim, with no control over your life and little responsibility. It would be worse if you were to deny the ADD and not take advantage of the help you could get, especially as employers and the legal system become more responsive to ADD and as treatment strategies become more effective.

This situation demands that you walk a certain kind of tightrope: doing your best, as if you could expect no help from anyone, yet accepting the help you do need to bring your life farther along. An extreme response would be either a fierce independence (accepting no help at all) or a chronic overindulgence (expecting the world to serve you because of your disability). The proper balance asks that you face your own sense of what is right and act accordingly. This might be a definition of integrity.

Don't Give Up

"Don't assume you're hopeless, even if you do have ADD," says Jeanette, a woman ADDer. "Even if these problems are genetic, it doesn't mean that you can't have any influence on them. You can." She also strongly advises adults with ADD to work on their self-esteem.

"Having ADD certainly makes a dent on one's self-esteem, but if you are honest with yourself and work hard at repairing the damage, you can make a big difference."

9

Common Mistakes Made by People Diagnosed with ADD

Let's say that you have been diagnosed with attention deficit disorder and you are currently undergoing treatment. The path ahead is now clear and your future is very bright, right? Unfortunately this is one of the common mistakes made by many people with ADD: Once diagnosed, they think their problems will magically disappear—and fast. This chapter discusses this and other common mistakes made by people with attention deficit disorder. Forewarned is forearmed!

Attitudinal Mistakes

After Diagnosis, Don't Expect a Miracle

After your ADD is diagnosed and treatment has begun, there is a good chance that your life will improve. However, many ADDers expect an instant cure when they start treatment.

"The toughest part after diagnosis and at the start of treatment is that we expect things will change drastically, but they don't," says Marie, a woman with ADD.

"Depression sets in for many as we realize we have to work at it. Usually not as hard as we used to—but then we expected miracles after being diagnosed."

Adults with moderate and severe ADD should begin medication, of course, if it is recommended by a skilled medical doctor. But they should also undertake psychotherapy with a mental health professional who specializes in ADD. Adds Marie, "People are often so caught up in their past experiences, feelings of rejection, feeling unsuccessful, feeling so different and out-of-it, that they really need to learn how to work through the past so that they can move on to the future."

Don't Expect the World to Suddenly Understand

Often when adults are diagnosed with ADD, they have an "aha" experience: They finally have an explanation for all those puzzling behaviors that people criticized them for. And they may be able to see possible solutions: medication and therapy, for example. This is a move in the right direction. But the mistake made by many adults with ADD is that they presume, once *they* have had their epiphany, that the rest of the world will understand. Over the years I have been working with various kinds of disabled people; and I must report, sadly, that the world tends *not* to understand.

"The hardest part for me was trying to make other people understand," says Connie, who is successfully coping with her ADD. "They just don't 'get' it. They still believe if I cared more or tried harder, and so forth, that things would be all right." She has become very frustrated trying to explain ADD to those who are close to her, along with what she feels to be others' failure to understand how it affects her.

Even though you try to educate people about ADD, they may not accept the diagnosis as legitimate. Step back rather than allow yourself to become stressed or annoyed. Once you've provided people with information, it is up to them to believe it or not. You know ADD is valid and real, but you cannot force other people to understand.

As more information about ADD is disseminated in the public sector and the media, we can hope that the general public—as well as mental health professionals and physicians—will grasp ADD and understand its dimensions.

Don't See ADD in Everyone

Mental health professionals report that a person who is diagnosed with ADD often suddenly notices that everyone has it: his or her spouse, boss, friends, next-door neighbor—everyone. But the person with ADD is not trained to evaluate or diagnose others; and as stated before, the diagnosis can even be difficult for a qualified and experienced mental health professional.

But this doesn't seem to stop many people, who, with their new enthusiasm, will assure their friends, family, and colleagues: "You are definitely ADD." What the ADDer sees in others may be everyday behavior, not a "disorder." For example, your boss locks himself out of his car, forgets where he put some important papers, and then says he'll delay the work that was due today. Inattentiveness, forgetfulness, and procrastination—all hallmarks of ADD, right? No.

You can't go by a person's behavior on one particular day, or even over the course of several weeks. What you may not know is that this man's wife blew up at him this morning. He is confused, upset, depressed, and distractible—all because of a problem he is facing. It could be that he *does* need professional counseling for ADD, but he may also need counseling to address his marital problem.

Even if you have known a person for a long time and think that he or she clearly has ADD, you could still be wrong because there are other problems he or she may face and not have told you about. Or he could have a psychiatric problem unrelated to ADD. Or maybe she really does have ADD! It's best not to tell a person that you are sure he has ADD. Instead, you might describe the symptoms of ADD; and if the person "sees" himself in these behaviors, then you can suggest that he seek an evaluation—and read this book.

People may also press you to tell them if they have ADD, but you need to resist. You should no more tell people that they have attention deficit disorder than you would tell them that they have diabetes or some other ailment. Let the professionals do the diagnosing!

Don't Blame All Your Problems on ADD

Another common mistake made by people with ADD is attributing all their mistakes and problems to it. "I forgot to turn in that report! Oh well, it's my ADD, so I can't help it." Although employers must make certain accommodations to the work environment if you ask them (but be careful with this), the world will not readily adapt to your ADD.

Thus if you blame everything on your ADD, you are using it as an excuse and a crutch. Some of your problems may have nothing to do with ADD at all. And if you feel you have no control, you are less likely to attempt to resolve the problems. So acknowledge your ADD, and realize that, with medication, therapy, and work on your own part, you can have a better life than you led before.

Medication-Related Mistakes

The First Medication Doesn't Help

Many people become discouraged when, after learning they have ADD, they take Ritalin (or Dexedrine or another drug for ADD) and their symptoms don't decrease at all. Or maybe they feel *worse*. They may think they are hopeless. Don't give up!

When physicians treat ADD, depression, and many other problems, it's a trial-and-error process. Because individual biochemistries vary and there are no biological tests to indicate an optimal level of medication (or even whether it's the "right" medication), doctors must have you try one medication at a time. The first one may not work—or the second or even the third.

Try to be patient. Most people will respond to one medication or a combination of medications. Certainly you should not give up if, after the first medication, you don't get good results. If you had an infection and the first antibiotic failed to clear it up, would you tell your doctor that you refuse to try another antibiotic? Would you be content to remain sick?

You Forgot Whether You Took Your Medication or Not

This is another classic problem for most ADDers. You are supposed to take a medicine that helps you remember things—but you forget whether or not you took it! Some people can tell if they haven't taken their medicine by how they feel. "I start to get a headache and I think, uh oh, I didn't take my medicine," says Cal. Others may feel "different," but they really aren't sure what to attribute it to. And they don't want to take too much medication: That could be dangerous.

So what do you do? You can try to link your pill taking to mealtimes if possible and if it is recommended—Ritalin is often taken on an empty stomach. Or you could set your watch to beep at a specific time for medication. Or buy a little pillbox at the pharmacy that requires you to put in a set number of pills for the day or week.

So when you aren't sure if you took your medicine, you can look at the pillbox: If the space is empty for that time of day, then you took your pill; if the pill is still in there, then you didn't.

Ask others in your ADD support group how they have tried to resolve this problem. Many people with ADD are extremely creative, and someone in your group may have found an ingenious solution.

Figure out a strategy that works for you. (Sometimes you will still forget, and you need to accept this fact.) Remember that ADD is, in part, a problem of dealing with time, a sort of temporal disability. But you can build structures into your life that will help you along.

Don't "Try" Your Child's Medication (or Your Spouse's or Friend's) and Don't Lend It Out Either

If your child has been diagnosed with ADD and is on medication that seems to improve his or her behavior, and you think that you also have ADD, you may be tempted to try one or two of your child's medications. Don't do it. Medications act differently on people within the same family, and what is effective for one person can make another person ill. And you could end up depriving your child of a needed medication.

It's far better to make an appointment with a physician and share your concerns. It takes more time, it costs money, but it's the right way to proceed. Also, don't give your medication to your spouse or friend for these or any other reasons. In addition, it is illegal.

Other Mistakes

One mistake many ADDers (and their significant others) make is to assume that all those old homilies they learned from their parents and society about how to concentrate and how to succeed are true: for example, the prevailing belief that a person always needs to sit at a desk in a quiet place in order to get work done. (Many teachers believe this of children with ADD, unfortunately.)

The truth is that complete quiet can irritate some people with ADD, and they may work *better* surrounded by noise and a jumble of activities. Some adults I have worked with report that they do well with the radio or television turned on in the background. If everything is turned off, they are straining to hear something—anything. But many do need total quiet.

Some people with ADD can use their computers on the train or plane and are oblivious to what's going on around them. This is partly hyperfocusing and partly a comfort level with background noise and tension. Their "desk" may be the airline tray table or their own laps, and that is fine. So, becoming aware of your own specific needs is a valuable part of your "program" to cope with ADD in your life.

There are probably many other mistaken assumptions made by adults with attention deficit disorder—and their friends and families. Let me know if any mistakes—especially the funny ones—stand out in sharp relief. And let me know your success stories too. Write to me. My address is listed in the postscript and in Appendix D.

10

Women with ADD

To date, most research on ADD has been done with boys and men. Girls and women were thought to suffer from ADD rarely, with the ratio of boys to girls at about 8 to 1. But in the past few years researchers have begun to find that many girls and women have gone undiagnosed. In a sense, they have been shortchanged by society and by the mental health profession.

How did this happen? From my professional perspective, let me assure you: Research in psychiatry is very difficult to do, for many reasons. One of the most important factors is having a sufficient number of research subjects. Since so many more boys than girls were thought to have ADD, it made perfect sense to study boys alone; otherwise the researcher would not have a large enough sample of people to study. Another difficulty is defining the disorder clearly. Since attention deficit disorder had always been associated with hyperactivity, that version of the disorder was the most obvious focus of study. ADD *without* hyperactivity was put on the back burner, even when it was noticed to be a problem. Besides, the quiet ADD child doesn't create demands on the school's resources, so why bother? Since hyperactivity is easier to define and there are more subjects available with this form of the disorder, research developed in this area.

As the scientific study of ADD has grown, more emphasis has been placed on the purely Inattentive Type of the disorder. And the sharpening of this focus has brought into the picture this question: Where have all the girls and women been? Perhaps females have a different type of ADD than the type prevalent among males. And they may suffer as much. This shift in focus might expand what we thought was true about ADD in general.

For these reasons, and because more than half of my adult ADD patients are women, I am devoting an entire chapter to women with ADD.

Other mental health professionals also report that about half of their adult ADD patients are female. Perhaps this is because women are more likely than men to seek counseling. But this still goes against the recent conventional wisdom that ADD boys and men outnumber ADD girls and women, anywhere from 4 to 10 males to 1 female.

Do Women "Get" ADD?

Because boys represent the overwhelming majority of the children who are diagnosed with ADD, it would appear to make sense that most adult ADDers are male. When researchers decided to look at former patients who are now adults, they were almost always boy children.

So it is not surprising that the predominant belief has been that ADD is a mostly male disorder. But maybe this belief is wrong. Scientists are now speculating that girls *do* have ADD, perhaps in about equal numbers with boys. But far too often the attention deficit disorder remains undiagnosed. There are several theories why this might be the case. Perhaps ADD shows up later in girls. Or maybe no one looked for ADD in girls—so people didn't find it. In a study of girls with attention deficit disorder reported in the November 1985 issue of *Pediatrics,* researchers stated, "ADD with hyperactivity is so widely accepted as a predominantly 'boys' disorder that there may be a failure to even consider the possibility of ADD with hyperactivity in girls and a consequent failure to identify all but the most severely affected girls" (Berry et al., 1985).

When something is not expected, it usually won't be perceived. Only very hyperactive girls would be noticed by teachers and clinicians because of the belief that girls just don't "get" ADD.

Or it could be related to a cultural issue. If a girl exhibits the dreamy, inattentive form of ADD and doesn't get in anybody's way, she probably won't be identified as having ADD. In other instances the bright girl or woman with ADD may be seen as someone with only average intelligence and abilities, primarily because limitations in her ability to pay attention do not allow her to achieve her potential.

Girls Are Generally Less Aggressive—and Aggression Gets Noticed

Experts have also found that there is a sort of "gender protection" for girls, and that girls must exhibit far more serious behavioral disorders than boys to be referred to mental health professionals. Also, fewer females with attention deficit disorder exhibit the aggression and conduct disorder that young males with ADD display. As a result Johnny, who is wreaking havoc, is far more likely to be referred to a pediatrician or psychiatrist for his "problem" than the distractible but quiet Janie.

In one of the few studies of females with ADD, reported in the *American Journal of Psychiatry* in January 1991 (Faraone et al.), researchers found that girls identified as having ADD had far greater problems with memory and learning, lower self-esteem, and were significantly more depressed than boys diagnosed with ADD.

Interestingly, the girls had a lower rate of acting out than the boys; and this factor alone may have been the key reason that clinicians have not identified girls as having ADD. Further, adult women with ADD are less likely than ADD men to exhibit aggressive or negative behavior. So when they seek help from a psychologist or psychiatrist, it's more likely that they will be diagnosed with depression, anxiety, or some problem other than attention deficit disorder.

The Underdiagnosis or Misdiagnosis of Women

Some experts speculate that many women are underdiagnosed because of cultural expectations. Authors John Ratey, Andrea Miller, and Kathleen Nadeau (in *A Comprehensive Guide to Attention Deficit Disorder in Adults*) have speculated that women may often be misdiagnosed: "The recognition of attentional problems and the diagnosis of ADD in women escapes even the best clinicians, because these women often lack the typical symptoms of hyperactivity and impulsivity in childhood or adulthood, and because the social filters through which we view women's behavior often are brought to bear upon our interpretation of symptoms."

As a result, women—if they are diagnosed at all—may be diagnosed with depression, anxiety disorder, perhaps even borderline personality disorder or phobias. According to these researchers, "the common clues we have guiding us toward diagnosis are not obvious, while other symptoms and co-morbid disorders serve to disguise the real problem. Yet, there the ADD still lurks, with its internal reality of restlessness, boredom, cognitive and affective impulsivity, disorganization and distractibility, and, of course, an inability to pay attention."

Several studies support this view. One 1994 study of people with ADD, reported in *Psychiatry Research,* revealed that women with ADD showed higher rates of anxiety disorder and major depression than a control group of women without ADD.

The researchers stressed the critical importance of diagnosing ADD, observing, "The underidentification and undertreatment of females with AD/HD may have substantial mental health and educational implications, suggesting that research is needed to develop a better understanding of AD/HD in females" (Biederman et al., 1994).

In another study (*Pediatric Neurology,* 1987), researchers found that some groups with ADD were overlooked by educators and others who identify children with ADD. The children in these groups succeeded by their wits and intense effort. Within the underidentified group, according to authors of the article, were girls with ADD:

> When we begin to compare boys and girls with ADD, we find that many of the clinical characteristics in girls are similar to those described for boys; however, there are several important differences. Girls with ADD have an increased frequency of cognitive and language deficits and increased social liability: that is, their relationships with their peers often are much more impaired than is the case in boys. Girls with ADD, however, exhibit far less physical aggression and loss of control. Because symptoms of aggression and loss of control usually bring ADD boys to medical attention, it is not surprising that girls with ADD represent an underidentified and underserved population which is at significant risk for academic, social, and emotional difficulties (Shaywitz and Shaywitz, 1987).

Children with unidentified ADD are more likely to be chided for undermotivation (seen as "not trying hard enough")—yet these children are actually struggling more than their peers. If this is true of children, then it seems likely that the unidentified girls—as well as unidentified boys—continue to have problems as adults. These patterns would likely continue into adulthood.

Since we now know that approximately half of the ADD children continue to show symptoms in adulthood, it is likely the same would be true of all the ADD girls we have been failing to diagnose over the years.

Families of Girls with ADD

Researchers have also looked at the families of ADD girls and boys and found that the relatives of the girls had higher rates of depression, anxiety, and other disorders than did the families of girls without ADD. This again suggests a genetic influence for ADD, similar to the genetic basis researchers have found in boys.

Author and therapist Sari Solden has looked at the issue of women with ADD in her book *Women with Attention Deficit Disorders: Embracing Disorganization at Home and in the Workplace.* Solden believes that women with ADD are much less likely than men to be hyperactive and, like the researchers mentioned earlier, she believes that women are far less likely to be diagnosed. She also assumes that "those who have gone undiagnosed the longest often have the most serious consequences." These consequences could include depression, substance abuse, very low self-esteem, chronic job failure, and other serious problems.

According to Solden, women in the Western world are expected to organize their own lives as well as the lives of others. When they cannot, they are seen as incompetent, uncaring, even bad. "Disorganization is especially significant for women, who are often expected to 'hold things together,'" she writes. "The symptom of disorganization is a major reason women cannot meet the cultural expectations of society."

The issue may be far simpler to understand if we recall that the ADD diagnosis has a long history of association with hyperactivity—ever since the earliest days of tracking this disorder. ADD has usually been associated with overt, active behavior. Only recently has the diagnosis included children and adults who had solely inattentive symptoms. So people with the inattentive form of ADD have been relatively neglected over the years.

In a way, this makes perfect sense. The active and troublesome boys do, in fact, demand more attention from researchers because they are the ones who are disrupting the classroom and sometimes getting into trouble. Of course, they also command the attention of mental health professionals. But this leaves behind all the inattentive types of ADD. And that category is where most of the girls might be found.

With a new understanding of the different kinds of ADD, girls and women may at last receive the professional help they need.

Problems with Medication

Because of cultural misunderstandings and physician misdiagnoses of women with ADD, women who seek treatment may be taking medications that do not help them. For example, the doctor may think a woman's hormones are the problem—it's PMS or maybe it's an early menopause. Or it's puberty. Or it's stress.

About twenty years ago the woman might have been given Valium, a powerful tranquilizer. Today she's more likely to be given Prozac, an antidepressant. The problem is that what she may really need is a stimulant such as Ritalin or Dexedrine. So she takes the Valium or Prozac. The woman may become tired, but the problem is not resolved. So she goes back to the physician and the doctor gives her some other tranquilizer or antidepressant. That doesn't work either.

Until mental health professionals and physicians accept attention deficit disorder as a "real" disorder and that women suffer from the problem, it will continue to exist. It doesn't have to be that way! And that is one reason why you are reading this book.

Sexuality and Women with ADD

As discussed earlier in this book, people with ADD may have trouble with hypo- or hypersexuality—and this is a significant issue for women with ADD. The woman who is hyposexual and resistant to touch may be seen as "cold" or even "frigid," while the hypersexual woman may be perceived as a "slut" or a "tramp." All of these labels carry a load of blame. Some mental health professionals may delve deeply into a woman's past seeking to identify some sexual abuse or traumatic event, when in fact her sexual problems stem from the undiagnosed ADD.

Compulsive or Impulsive Behavior

Society also frowns on the woman who "shops until she drops" or who rushes out on some sudden impulse. Instead, the married woman with children is expected to be a good wife and mother, although today it is culturally acceptable (if not expected) for the woman to have an outside job.

Reactions to Cultural Norms

When a woman cannot comply with cultural norms—for example, she maintains a messy house with boxes or piles everywhere—society frowns on her, and the woman internalizes this censure. She may feel shame and guilt. She may periodically attempt a massive clean sweep of her home, but the mess quickly piles up again.

Or what if the undiagnosed woman with ADD is working on a project she loves and she forgets to pick up her child at school? If this happens more than once, she is condemned as a "bad mother." The problem is that this behavior will probably continue unless the woman receives treatment. After hearing again and again that she is a bad mother, her emotional pain will be great.

Much worse, if the woman is engaged in numerous love affairs or if she becomes a substance abuser, society may actually regard her as bad, particularly if she is a caregiver to children.

As an undiagnosed ADD woman ages, she is more likely to experience guilt, shame, and anxiety if some of these negative behavior patterns persist. And it becomes even more urgent for her to receive treatment.

The ADD Mom

One area in which a woman with ADD may really have a problem is parenting. Society still envisions the mother as the key parent, and when she "falls down on the job," it is considered terrible indeed. If the mom with ADD has a *child* with ADD, the problem is exacerbated. Even if both Dad and Mom have ADD, who is more likely to get blamed for failing to do some child-related task? Mom.

For example, let's say a child forgets to do his homework and is generally having trouble in school. The teacher may meet with the mom and encourage her to help the child organize his work, put it in special folders, and so forth. But what if the ADD mother is disorganized and distractible herself, and if she forgets to help her child to do what's been asked or fails to encourage him because she's thinking about something else?

Eventually the ADD mom will be seen as a "bad mother." After all, why isn't she helping her own child? What's the matter with her?

What's the matter with her may well be the same as what is the matter with her child—only the mother may have gone undiagnosed. Let's change the scenario so that the mother *is* diagnosed. Now the mother can explain to the teacher that she, too, has ADD, that it's hard for her to organize, but that she will work on it. Then the mother can write herself notes—for example on a whiteboard—to "help Jimmy with homework—4 P.M." She can also create other interventions, as described elsewhere in this book. The entire situation would be much improved if the mother realized that she had ADD and received appropriate treatment.

The Wife of the ADD Husband

There is another woman who needs attention. She is the *wife* of the man with attention deficit disorder. Often she has been the one who managed much of her husband's life, making sure he had his briefcase, keys, and other necessary paraphernalia and helping him find things when he loses them. He may have had a secretary who handled such details at work and a wife at home to manage his home life.

But the 1950s view of Mom at home baking brownies while Dad is at work is long gone, and now most women also work outside the home. No longer are they picking up the pieces that the man with ADD leaves behind.

As women play less of a "cleanup" role, men may find themselves having to pick up the ball—literally! As a result, men with ADD may find themselves more vulnerable than ever because of their inability to get organized without some kind of outside help.

This does *not* mean that it is the woman's "fault" that boys and men are so frequently diagnosed with ADD. Rather, if we acknowledge that some men and some women have ADD, and that changing societal roles have affected both genders, then we can better deal with the problem.

When the ADD Woman Is Married to the ADD Man

Sometimes a woman with ADD is married to a man who also has ADD—and without treatment, watch out! It might even be that they were attracted to each other because of their ADD qualities. No other person could understand them! It is also possible that such a relationship will work out without professional help. If the couple recognizes their problem, they can avoid a breakup as well as problems in their work lives. The good news is that treatment and hard work can help a lot.

Conclusion

It seems clear that girls and many women in our society could be underdiagnosed or misdiagnosed, which can cause many problems for these women, their families, and society in general. If you are a woman and think you have ADD, but have been diagnosed with depression or another problem, ask your mental health professional to reevaluate you or seek a second opinion. Maybe you don't have ADD, but it's a diagnosis that should at least be considered if you feel you fit the profile described in this book.

Postscript

100 Bites of Advice for the Rushed, Impatient, Harried, and Distractible

What would a book on adult ADD be if it didn't have a bunch of bite-sized suggestions that you can read when you don't have time to read anything? Many of the tips on this list are taken from this book. Some are borrowed from other writers in the field. Some I heard somewhere but forget where. Some are my own, and I've used them with patients over the years. I know that I'm not the only one who makes these kinds of lists. But you don't often find 100 bites of advice in one place.

1. *Never Give Up*.
2. Keep your own counsel. Well-meaning advice from someone else may not be good for you.
3. Keep track of some behavior that indicates how you are doing *(behavioral markers)*. If you forget, pick it up again. Make a chart and note when the interventions were started.
4. Have as many handles on happiness as you can (from Jane Austen).
5. If in doubt about how to interpret a situation, let it be positive. If you are going to make your-

self miserable, at least have good evidence that things are really bad. (Most situations in life are ambiguous, which means that they can be viewed as positive.)

6. Do random acts of kindness.

7. Each day do one thing that is difficult but good for you to do. It builds character (from William James).

8. Give out compliments liberally, especially if you are the ADD type who needs to work on social skills.

9. When you say hello to someone, smile.

10. When you greet someone, liberally use phrases such as "How are you?" or "How was your weekend/trip?" It doesn't mean too much, but it greases the wheels.

11. Wave at fire trucks. It engenders innocent fun— but only one wave per truck!

12. Clean up your diet; it may help. Eliminate chocolate, sugar, desserts, coffee, soda, alcohol, and go very light on red meat.

13. Recognize the positive aspects of ADD, especially the energy, creativity, and liveliness.

14. Support groups can be very comforting and informative, but they are not likely to do the whole job in your treatment.

15. Get a *clutter buddy* if you need one. You could do the same thing with regard to goals—find what could be called a *goal buddy*.

16. Listen to doctors carefully, but don't worship them. Even God gives us free choice.

17. Use *composing moments*. Let yourself gather your thoughts and see where you need to

refocus. This takes a short time—a minute or two, maybe five.

18. Spend 15 to 30 minutes each day confronting your clutter. Become friendly with it.

19. Consider hiring a *professional organizer* if you can afford it. It will speed up your clutter management.

20. Consider developing the practice of meditation.

21. Be open-minded about medication. It was created for a reason.

22. Vigorous, regular exercise is recommended by some ADD experts. Consult with your doctor before starting an exercise program.

23. Throw out or donate belongings you don't use anymore. Free yourself of clutter.

24. Having a *coach* is valuable. Talking on the phone daily with an objective person may help you to focus and manage your time better.

25. Make frequent use of lists. Spend time every day working on it.

26. An electronic organizer can be set to remind you of the various things you need to do. Such prompts are good helpers. An organizer also helps you to remember your afternoon medication.

27. External aids are helpful for many ADD people because otherwise they might forget what they have to do. Use signs, Post-Its, and whiteboards at home and at the workplace, along with alarms on your organizer, watch, or timer.

28. Try to handle mail and other papers only once (OHIO = Only Handle It Once).

29. Transition times, changing from one activity to another, may be harder for ADD people. So

give yourself more time. Call it *collecting and changing time.*

30. Use pencil and paper to work out some problems. The external reality can be remarkably clarifying.

31. Break down tasks and projects into smaller steps. Use pencil and paper. Copy over your chart and make it look nice.

32. Use color coding as a way to help you organize—colored folders, notes, Post-Its. It's also more fun.

33. Use a *work board* or bulletin board to organize your tasks and projects. And different colors too (see Viscott's *Action Board.*)

34. You may never understand your ADD completely. That's the way most things are in life. It's okay.

35. Use 6 alarm clocks—if you have to—in order to get up on time.

36. Plan your day the night before.

37. Having a person with you may be all you need to do something you have been avoiding, such as cleaning up your clutter. Ask the person not to talk.

38. Use 5 minutes each hour to compose yourself and refocus your energies.

39. Timers can help keep you on track. Ticking ones drive me nuts. I prefer digital.

40. Have a *quiet time* each day to do your paperwork. Screen your phone calls and take only emergencies. Close your door. Let others know about this routine.

41. Your time may be valuable. Learn to delegate routine tasks to others.

42. Make eye contact with people when you talk to them. They will feel you're listening. But don't stare.

43. Knowing your diagnosis is better than not knowing—for most people. Keep at it until you learn the truth.

44. Help others with ADD, especially if you sense they need support or knowledge. It feels good.

45. But don't become an evangelist.

46. Work with the book *Feeling Good,* by David Burns, to help correct your negative thinking. Do the written exercises because they will help you improve *much* faster.

47. If your social relationships are not what you would like them to be, consider group therapy. If you can't find an ADD group, join another, but stay in it for at least 18 months. You can't see your own social flaws; you need to spend a lot of time in a group to get at them.

48. Give yourself rewards for a job well done. Most people don't know our struggles, so we may have to pat ourselves on the back.

49. Keep the desk clear if you can. It will help to reduce distractions.

50. Simplify your life—your living space, belongings, relationships. But you may need stimulation to get yourself to do things: watch out for this tendency.

51. Be careful about getting into *organizer mania*— using a Day Runner, an electronic organizer, to-do lists galore, becoming a pain-in-the-neck neatnik. You could become insufferable.

52. Do not build a case against yourself. Minimize self-blame or downing yourself. All of the great

spiritual teachers in history have pointed out how imperfect we all are. And it's still okay. That's the way life was designed.

53. Eliminate the necessity of perfectionism in your life, if you lean in that direction. As Albert Ellis, a renowned psychologist, points out, "Anything in life is worth doing in a mediocre way." Dr. Ellis sometimes has people do deliberately ridiculous things so that they can get over the pressure of having to do everything just right.

54. Structure your time so that the stress of making decisions can be reduced. For example, Monday nights are set aside for studying X and Y, Tuesdays from 7 to 10 P.M. is for Z, and so on.

55. Plan your activities to conform with your goals. (Simple—but who actually goes over this carefully?)

56. To work on reducing social intrusiveness, try to imagine a person encircled in a Hula Hoop, which signifies the person's private space (from Kelly and Ramundo).

57. Establish a rule of no arguments at the dinner table.

58. Try to systematize the time you go to bed and wake up in the morning: make it the same, and reasonable, time each day.

59. Don't expect others to truly understand you. Hardly anyone will "get it."

60. Develop *anchor places* and *anchor points* in your life so that your things will have a home and your time will be structured by healthy routines.

61. Map out driving routes before leaving on a car trip.

62. Developing public-speaking skills is a powerful way to enhance your self-esteem.

63. Be aware that, even with the best treatment, it is likely that your ADD will not go away. But you will probably be in better shape, be better informed, and you will know your strengths and weaknesses. Treatment can give you a *tool kit* of coping strategies to help you in times of trouble. These 100 tips offer a few of them.

64. Classical music, particularly Mozart and Bach, is very beneficial for many people's moods. I personally believe that this music is healing.

65. Think of mistakes as important information—from which you have learned something.

66. Clothes that have not been worn for the last year should be donated. Donate books too.

67. Get nice storage containers to help yourself with organizing; they will also make the process more fun.

68. Use *between times*—commercials on TV, waiting in line, commuting—to take care of small tasks, such as writing checks, copying addresses, writing a thank-you note (see tip 89).

69. Don't—*don't, don't*—try to follow all of these tips. Too much! Try one and see if you can work on it. Then move on.

70. Background music can help some people to focus better. Sound machines (white noise) also work for some people.

71. Keep a journal. Note your progress, and especially your successes. Consider writing down *only* your successes if your self-esteem needs a boost.

72. Use the ABC method of prioritizing tasks for

the day: A = must do; B = important; C = can wait. Use paper and pencil or pen. Check things off when they're done. I use 3×5 cards that fit in my shirt pocket.

73. When you structure your time, weave in pleasurable events to look forward to, and use them as reinforcers.

74. When you read something fairly important, take notes. This will help you stay connected to the material.

75. *"What is the best use of my time right now?"* Ask yourself this question frequently.

76. Consider asking a friend to let you know when you drift off in a social situation (in privacy, after the event of course).

77. Mornings are often fuzzy times for many ADD people. Don't plan important or high-concentration events in the morning, and plan something pleasurable at this time so that you'll be encouraged to get out of bed.

78. Taking notes can be a way to keep your attention on a speaker, even if you never refer to them again.

79. If impulsivity is a problem, make it a focus of your journal. Note the times you are impulsive and try to discern what happened to trigger the impulsive behavior. This will make you more conscious of a pattern in your impulsiveness. A therapist is also usually good at discerning such patterns. But leave a space on the page where you noted the impulsive behavior. A few days later rewrite the "script" to portray what you would have liked to happen. This programs the positive script into your brain.

80. If you find yourself talking too much in a social situation, just pause after finishing a sentence and leave some "air time" for the other person. Ask a simple question to draw in the other person. Memorize a few such questions ahead of time.

81. Never criticize, condemn, or complain (from Dale Carnegie). If you can follow this advice, I'm impressed!

82. Finish one project before starting another.

83. Learn how to admit your mistakes. This makes you a person of integrity. It also feels good—in a certain odd way.

84. If you have trouble *appearing* to be listening, rephrase the last thing said by the other person as a way of keeping yourself connected to the person to whom you're speaking. This is an old counseling technique of the renowned psychologist Carl Rogers.

85. Take a walk-around break to work off your energy. Flex your muscles if you sit a lot. Try sit-ups in the middle of the day if you can manage it physically.

86. When you are planning your day, give yourself more time than you think you need to do tasks. Adding an extra 50 percent is a common rule of thumb.

87. Watch out for overcommitment, very common in the enthusiastic ADD person. Think before you say yes. In fact, delay any commitment for at least a day: "Let me think about it" is a good line.

88. Develop a series of socially acceptable questions that you can ask when at a party—for example,

"How do you know Sally?" "Are you in the same profession as David?" "What do you think of the (latest political/current event)?"

89. You can compensate for seeming to be inattentive by doing some extra-attentive things, such as sending a card to a person who has done something nice for you, giving very thoughtful gifts, allowing the other person to be the first to get out of an elevator or door.

90. Arrange tasks so that the *pleasant* event follows the *less pleasant* event. This is called the *Premack principle.* For example, you could arrange a whole series of events or tasks in such a way that each event in the series is more pleasant than the one that preceded it.

91. When organizing your home, arrange your things into three categories: "never use," "sometimes use," and "actively use." Put the first category of boxes in the basement or some other storage place. Or take the leap and throw it away—or donate it (from Kelly and Ramundo).

92. Utilize *stimulus control:* To minimize distractions, set up your study place or desk with *only* those things needed in that environment and for your specific purpose. Then *use* that space only for its designated purpose: Don't study on your bed, don't eat at your desk.

93. Finances are often troublesome for ADD adults. Write down everything you spend. And . . .

94. Minimize credit cards.

95. Practice frugality.

96. Put 10 percent of your income away in savings.

Dip into it *only* in an emergency—a *real* emergency.

97. Avoid television.

98. Avoid rush hour if you can.

99. Don't become obsessed with your ADD, especially as an excuse for your failings. And don't convert your disorder into some kind of *mission*. That can be obnoxious. Besides, there are already too many of us doing that. It's getting crowded in here.

100. A phrase that is comforting to many: *Be still, and know that I am God* (Psalm 46).

Concluding Remarks

Maybe you have learned that you might have attention deficit disorder, and you've made that first appointment to see a mental health professional. Congratulations! It won't necessarily be an easy path, but you are now on the road to improving your life.

There will be naysayers and scoffers who say that ADD is a made-up ailment for lazy people. You know they're wrong, and so do increasing numbers of educators, mental health professionals, and the general public. You can try to educate them about differences in the brains of people with ADD and their differing biochemistries. But there are people who just won't get it.

Don't worry about them! Just hold your head up high and know that ADD is a *real* problem with real solutions. They're out there. I hope this book will give you a head start down the road to a better life.

* * *

If you would like to share your thoughts or any information about attention deficit disorder among adults with me, I am interested in hearing from you. I am especially interested in your success stories. Write to me or send electronic mail to: Dr. J. L. Thomas, Director, NeuroServices, Inc., 19 West 34th Street, Penthouse, New York, NY 10001. E-mail: nurosvcs@aol.com.

And never give up!

Appendix A: Keeping Track of My Progress*

Instructions: Score yourself each week—0 for no problem, 1 for a mild problem, 2 for a moderate problem, and 3 for significant problems. Provide this information to your mental health professional.

1. *Inattention*

   a. Fails to give close attention to details or makes careless mistakes in schoolwork, work, or other activities

   b. Often has difficulty sustaining attention in tasks

   c. Often does not seem to listen to what is being said

   d. Often does not follow through on instructions and fails to perform duties in the workplace (not due to failure to understand instructions)

   e. Often has difficulties organizing tasks and activities

* Criteria used from *DSM-IV*

WEEK 1   WEEK 2   WEEK 3   WEEK 4   WEEK 5   WEEK 6

____   ____   ____   ____   ____   ____

____   ____   ____   ____   ____   ____

____   ____   ____   ____   ____   ____

____   ____   ____   ____   ____   ____

____   ____   ____   ____   ____   ____

f. Often avoids or strongly dislikes tasks (such as those that require sustained mental effort)

g. Often loses things necessary for tasks or activities

h. Often easily distracted by extraneous stimuli

i. Often forgetful in daily activities.

2. *Hyperactivity-Impulsivity*

a. Often fidgets with hands or feet or squirms in seat

b. Leaves seat in situations when remaining seated is expected

c. Often has difficulty engaging in leisure activities quietly

d. Often blurts out answers to questions before the questions have been completed

e. Often has difficulty waiting in line or awaiting turn in group situations

Week 1	Week 2	Week 3	Week 4	Week 5	Week 6
_____	_____	_____	_____	_____	_____
_____	_____	_____	_____	_____	_____
_____	_____	_____	_____	_____	_____
_____	_____	_____	_____	_____	_____
_____	_____	_____	_____	_____	_____
_____	_____	_____	_____	_____	_____
_____	_____	_____	_____	_____	_____
_____	_____	_____	_____	_____	_____
_____	_____	_____	_____	_____	_____

Instructions: In this chart, list your behavioral markers—for example, losing things, forgetting tasks, and so forth—and rate yourself. It's okay to list less than five behavioral markers.

My Behavioral Markers

What They Are

1. _____
2. _____
3. _____
4. _____
5. _____

How I'm Doing

	WEEK 1	WEEK 2	WEEK 3	WEEK 4	WEEK 5	WEEK 6
Behavior 1	___	___	___	___	___	___
Behavior 2	___	___	___	___	___	___
Behavior 3	___	___	___	___	___	___
Behavior 4	___	___	___	___	___	___
Behavior 5	___	___	___	___	___	___

Appendix B: National Organizations

The ADDed Line
3790 Loch Highland Parkway
Roswell, GA 30339
800-982-4028

Adult ADD Association
1225 East Sunset Drive
Suite 640
Bellingham, WA 98226-3529
360-647-6681

Association on Higher Education and Disability
(AHEAD)
P.O. Box 21192
Columbus, OH 43221-0192
614-488-4972

Attention Deficit Disorder Association (ADDA)
P.O. Box 488
West Newbury, MA 01985

Attention Deficit Information Network, Inc.
475 Hillside Avenue
Needham, MA 02194
617-455-9895

Attention Deficit Resource Center
P.O. Box 71223
Marietta, GA 30007-1223

Children and Adults with Attention Deficit Disorder
(CH.A.D.D.)
499 NW 70th Avenue, Suite 308
Plantation, FL 33317
305-587-3700

Higher Education and Adult Training for People with
Handicaps (HEATH)
National Clearinghouse on Post-Secondary Education
for Handicapped Individuals
One Dupont Circle NW, Suite 800
Washington, DC 20036-1193
800-939-9320

Learning Disabilities Association
4156 Library Road
Pittsburgh, PA 15234
412-341-1515

LifeCoach
124 Waterman Street
Providence, RI 02906
800-253-4965
508-252-4965

The National Association of Professional Organizers
1033 LaPosada Drive, Suite 220
Austin, TX 78752-3880
512-206-0151

National Center for Law and Learning Disabilities
(NCLLD)
P.O. Box 368
Cabin John, MD 20818
301-469-8308

The National Coaching Network
P.O. Box 353
Lafayette Hill, PA 19444
610-825-4505
(Send $3 for an information packet)

The Personal and Professional Coaches Association
(PPCA)
P.O. Box 2838
San Francisco, CA 94126
415-522-8789

Professional Group for ADD and Related Disorders
(PGARD)
28 Fairview Road
Scarsdale, NY 10583

Rebus Institute
1499 Bayshore Boulevard, Suite 146
Burlingame, CA 94010
415-697-7424

Appendix C: National Newsletters

ADDed Line
3790 Loch Highland Parkway
Roswell, GA 30339

ADDendum
c/o CPS
5041-A Back Lick Road
Annandale, VA 22003
(An excellent newsletter, founded by Paul Jaffe.
Reviews of research, personal tips and stories,
new support groups, and conferences.)

ADDult News
c/o Mary Jane Johnston
ADDult Support Network
2620 Ivy Place
Toledo, OH 43613

CH.A.D.D.E.R.
(published by CH.A.D.D.)
499 Northwest 70th Avenue, Suite 308
Plantation, FL 33317

(CH.A.D.D. has only recently become a resource for adults with ADD.)

Challenge
P.O. Box 448
West Newbury, MA 01985
published by ADDA
(Has published interesting interviews.)

The Rebus Institute Report
1499 Bayshore Boulevard, Suite 146
Burlingame, CA 94010

Appendix D: Support Groups and Professional Help for ADD Adults

I have attempted to list only groups that deal with adult ADD and to exclude groups that focus on ADD children.

Contact CH.A.D.D. at their toll-free number, 800-233-4050, to find the chapter nearest you if this listing does not include one in your area. Be sure to tell them that you are primarily interested in a support group for adults.

Alaska
Anchorage CH.A.D.D.
907-338-1491

Arizona
Adults Seeking Knowledge About ADD
Steven Ledingham
520-749-5465
Ledingham@tikal.biosci.arizona or
Ledingham@aol.com
Also, http://128.196.15.4

Attention Deficit Disorder Clinic (Phoenix area)
602-863-7950

Attention Deficit Disorder Clinic (Scottsdale area)
602-423-7770

Center for Attention Deficit and Learning Disorders
(Paradise)
Sanford Silverman, Ph.D.
602-990-4474

Della Mays, Adult Coordinator
(Tucson)
602-887-0978

Families with Attention Deficit Disorder
Adult Group
(Chino Valley)
Marcia T. Brehmer
520-636-5160

South Mountain CH.A.D.D.
(Phoenix)
Jeri Goldstein, M.C.R.N.
602-345-6622

California
Adult Attention Deficit Disorder Group
(Arcadio)
Melissa Thomasson, Ph.D.
818-301-7977

Joan Andrews, L.E.P., M.F.C.C.
(Newport Beach)
714-476-0991

Patreen Bower, M.S., M.F.C.C.
Sue Griffith, M.A.
(Santa Ana)
714-953-8220

John Capel, Ph.D.
(Sacramento)
916-488-5788

CH.A.D.D. of Alameda County
(Hayward)
Kathy Schnepple
510-581-9941

CH.A.D.D. of the Conejo Valley
Kay Gilmore
805-520-4943

CH.A.D.D. of Mid-Peninsula
(Mountain View)
Kayleen Shorago
415-969-6233

Pat and Monte Churchill
(Pacheco)
510-825-4938

David Hayes, Adult Coordinator
(Tiburon)
415-435-0994

Milton Lucius, Ph.D.
(El Dorado Hills)
916-933-5217

MATRIX
(San Rafael)
415-499-3877

Karen Neale, M.A.
(Los Gatos)
408-395-1348

Kitty Petty ADD/LD Institute
(Mountain View)
415-969-7137

San Diego Support Group for Adults with Attention
Deficit Disorder
Amy Ellis
Roland Rotz, Ph.D.
Learning Development Services
619-276-6912

Colorado
CH.A.D.D. of Colorado Springs
719-597-9857

John Cizman
(Boulder)
303-786-8112

Maxine Jarvi
(Fort Collins)
970-223-1338

Don Lambert
(Arvada)
303-424-5272

Harry Orr
(Denver)
303-458-5675

Dennis Smith
(Littleton)
303-790-2354

Connecticut
Block & Stein/A.D.D. Associates
(Avon)
Dr. Ron Weinstein, Ph.D.
860-677-2926

CH.A.D.D. of the Farmington Valley
(West Simsbury)
860-651-3880

Liz Johnson, Cocoordinator
(Moodus)
203-873-1733

Paul Kalajain, Adult Coordinator
(Storrs)
203-487-1920

John Shusman
(Wethersfield)
203-257-3221

Delaware
Lizbee Mahoney, Adult Coordinator
CH.A.D.D. of Brandywine Valley
(Wilmington)
302-478-8202

Florida
CH.A.D.D. ADDult Group
(Orlando)
407-263-4222

CH.A.D.D. of Duval County
(Jacksonville)
904-390-0866

CH.A.D.D. Hillsborough/Polk County Chapter
(Tampa)
813-882-5310

CH.A.D.D. of South Broward/North Dade
(Cooper City)
Lora Mills
954-680-0799

Bethann Vetter, Adult Coordinator
(Jacksonville)
904-731-7230

Georgia
Adult Attention Deficit Disorder Support Group
(Decatur)
John Teach, Ph.D.
404-378-6643

L.D. Adults of Georgia
(Marietta)
Helene Johnson
770-514-8088

Illinois
ADD-ONS, Ltd.
(Frankfort)
Mary Daum, President
815-469-8567

Adult ADD Support Group
(Bloomington)
Ron Ropp, Rel.D.
309-829-0751

Deborah Dornaus
(Peoria)
309-693-0038

Gary Hubbard, M.S., L.M.F.T.
(Lowes Park)
815-282-1800

Indiana
Abilities Unlimited
(Bloomington)
Julia Dadds
812-332-1620

ADDults of Central Indiana
(Anderson)
317-649-2871

Teresa Gross
(Valparaiso)
219-465-0447

Ed Morris
(Noblesville)
317-773-9459

David Shultz
(South Bend)
219-232-6690

Iowa
Don Walker, Adult Coordinator
(Iowa City)
319-337-5201

Kansas
ADD/ADHD Education and Resource Association
(Prairie Village)
913-362-6108

Adult ADD Clinic
(Overland Park)
Avner Stern
(913) 469-6510

Kentucky
Nancy Blakley, Adult Coordinator
(Lexington)
606-223-3074

Louisiana
River Parish CH.A.D.D.
(Kenner)
Wanda Bardwell-Seiffert
504-467-4983

Maine
Lindy Botto
(Scarborough)
207-883-2528

Maryland
Montgomery County CH.A.D.D.
(Gaithersburg)
301-869-3628

Massachusetts
Linda Greenwood
(Plymouth)
508-747-2179

Linda Harrison
(Danvers)
508-777-4077

North Shore Adults and Children with ADD
(Lynn)
617-599-6818

Lori Ray, Adult Coordinator
(Greenfield)
413-773-5545

Michigan
Adult ADDvocacy
Fred Michaelson
810-380-0144

Adult ADD Awareness
(Sterling Heights)
Kathleen Van Howe
810-939-1112

Adult ADD Support Group
(Lansing)
Jennifer Bramer
517-483-1184

ADDult Information Exchange Network
(Ann Arbor)
Jim Reisinger
313-426-1659

Minnesota
Adult ADD Support Group
(Minnetonka)
William Ronan, LICSW
612-933-3460

Missouri
Attention Deficit Disorder Association of Missouri
(St. Louis)
Barb Rosenfeld, Adult Coordinator
314-963-4655

DePaul Health Center/Adults with ADD Support
Group
(Bridgeton)
314-344-7224

Montana
CH.A.D.D. of the Flathead Valley
(Kalispell)
Stephanie Luehr
406-756-6159

New Hampshire
Adult ADD Support Group
(Concord)
Sarah Brophy, Ph.D.
603-226-6121

White Mountain AD-IN (Adult)
(North Conway)
Joanne Duncan
603-356-2714

New Jersey
Adult ADD Support Group
(Red Bank)
Robert LoPresti, Ph.D.
908-842-4553

New Mexico
Attention Deficit Disorder Clinic
(Albuquerque)
Robert Gurnee
505-243-9600
505-820-1339

New York
CH.A.D.D. of Mohawk Valley
(Utica)
Janice Hall
315-724-4233

CH.A.D.D. of Westchester County
(Brewster)
914-278-3020

Greater Rochester Attention Deficit Disorder
Association (GRADDA)
(Rochester)
716-251-2322

NeuroServices, Inc.
J. Lawrence Thomas, Ph.D., Director
19 West 34th Street, Penthouse,
New York, NY 10001
212-268-8900

S. G. Salit, M.S.W., Adult Coordinator
(Scarsdale)
914-472-2935

Charlotte Tomaino, Ph.D.
(White Plains)
914-949-4055

Ohio
A.S.K. About ADD
(Spring Valley)
Bettylou Huber
513-862-4573

Oklahoma
Helping ADDults in Tulsa (HADD-IT)
Shelley Curtis
918-622-1370

Oregon
ADDVENTURES Support Group
(Portland)
503-452-5666

Pennsylvania
The Hahnemann Hospital Adult ADD Support
Group
(Lafayette Hill)
Susan Sussman, M.Ed.
610-825-8572

Main Line CH.A.D.D.
(Philadelphia suburbs)
610-626-2998

Southwest Pennsylvania CH.A.D.D. Network Adult
ADD Support Group
(Dormont)
412-531-4554

Rhode Island
Rhode Island ADDult Support Group
(Warwick)
Austin Donnelly
401-463-8778

South Carolina
Adult ADD Support Group
(Columbia)
Ron A. Ralph
c/o Mental Health Association in Mid-Carolina
803-733-5415

Tennessee
ADD's Up
(Nashville)
615-292-5947

Texas
ADHD and LD Support Group
(Houston)
512-477-5516

Central Houston Chapter for ADD/ADHD Adults
Chris Kipple
713-521-2420

Dallas Chapter for ADD/ADHD Adults
Melissa Petty
214-458-9226

North Houston Chapter for ADD/ADHD Adults
Karen Kasper
713-353-3898

North Texas CH.A.D.D.
Paul Jurek
817-383-5795
Sharon Montagne
817-566-0710

West Houston Chapter for ADD/ADHD Adults
Katrina Ricketts
713-870-0191

Utah
L.D.A. of Utah
(Salt Lake City)
Joyce Otterstrom
801-355-2881

Virginia
Adult Attention Deficit & Related Disorders
Outreach
(Newport News)
Jody Lochmiller
804-930-1931

Arlington/Alexandria CH.A.D.D.
703-536-6846

CH.A.D.D. of Central Virginia
(Richmond)
804-254-0124

Charlottesville CH.A.D.D.
804-979-5771

Harrisonburg/Rockingham CH.A.D.D.
540-289-6661

Northern Virginia Adult ADD Support Group
Susan Biggs, Ed.D.
703-641-5451

Peninsula Attention Deficit Disorder Association
(PADDA)
804-591-9119

Potomac of Virginia CH.A.D.D.
Maggie Baker
703-979-0820
Linda Earl
703-536-6846

Tidewater CH.A.D.D.
804-430-3673

Washington
ADDult Support of Washington
(Tacoma)
Cynthia Hammer
206-752-0801

ADDult Support of Washington for Adults with ADD
206-759-5085

Adult ADD Association
(Bellingham)
Lisa Poast
360-647-6681

Attention Deficit Disorder Clinic
(Olympia)
360-754-4801

Kathy Van Dyke
(Kennowick)
509-586-4257

Wisconsin
Adult ADHD Support Group
ADHD Women's Support Group
(Waukesha)
Paul Rembas
414-542-6694

Robert Lintereur
(Theinsville)
414-242-5387

Outside the United States
CH.A.D.D. Canada, Inc.
1376 Bank Street, Suite 214
Ottawa, Ontario, Canada
K1H 7H3
613-731-1209

CH.A.D.D. Vancouver Chapter
604-222-4043

Hyperactivity/Attention Deficit Association (N.S.W.)
29 Bertram Street
Chatswood 2067
Australia

Appendix E: On-line Resources

On-line (Computer) Support and Information Groups

The ADD Forum
CompuServe
If on-line, type GO ADD
Call CompuServe at 800-524-3388

ADD Group on America Online: Use the keyword
PEN to get to message boards, software libraries, etc.
For more information, send E-mail to Imroman
Call America Online at 800-827-6364.

Internet Listings

ADA [Americans with Disabilities Act] and Disability
Information
http://www.public.iastate.edu/~sbilling/ada.html

Adults Seeking Knowledge About ADD
http://128.196.15.4

Attention Deficit Disorder Archives
http://homepage.seas.upenn.edu/~mengwong/add/

Children and Adults with Attention Deficit Disorder
(CH.A.D.D.)
http://www.chadd.org

CyberPsychLink
http://cctr.umkc.edu/user/dmartin/psych2.html

Lifeworks (coaching organization)
http://www.kwik-linkl/com/kwik-link/c/lifeworks.html

National Alliance for the Mentally Ill (NAMI) ADD
Information
http://www.cais.com/vikings/mani/index.html

One ADD Place
http://www.greatconnectcom/oneaddplace/

Usenet group: alt.support.attn-deficit

Recommended Books and Other Resources

Books

Barkley, Russell, Ph.D. *Attention Deficit Hyperactivity Disorder*. New York: Guilford Press, 1990.

Although this is an academic (and dense) book, it is a standard in the field. Much of the book is about ADD in children. Barkley is a superb lecturer, and he is worth traveling to hear.

Hallowell, Edward M., M.D.; and Ratey, John J., M.D. *Driven to Distraction*. New York: Pantheon, 1994.

This book is an excellent overview of attention deficit disorder in adults and also includes material on children. Doctors Hallowell and Ratey are experienced psychiatrists in Cambridge, Massachusetts, and they are both ADD themselves. They might be the most skilled psychopharmacologists in the field.

Kelly, Kate; and Ramundo, Peggy, *You Mean I'm Not Lazy, Stupid or Crazy?! A Self-Help Book for Adults with Attention Deficit Disorder*. Cincinnati: Tyrell and Jerem Press, 1993.

This book, written by two adults with ADD, was one of the first books intended for ADD adults. It includes many practical and helpful hints.

Nadeau, Kathleen G., Ph.D. *A Comprehensive Guide to Attention Deficit Disorder in Adults*. New York: Brunner/Mazel, 1995.
This book includes essays by experts and provides broad coverage of research on ADD to date. Although geared toward the professional, it is not too difficult for anyone who is serious about gaining knowledge of the field. It contains some interesting chapters.

Weiss, Gabrielle, Ph.D.; and Hechtman, Lily Trokenberg, Ph.D. *Hyperactive Children Grown Up: ADHD in Children, Adolescents, and Adults*. New York: Guilford Press, 1993.
This book summarizes the research in the field, particularly the authors' studies of ADD children who are now young men. This is a dense book aimed at the academic community; but it is first-rate.

Weiss, Lynn, Ph.D. *Attention Deficit Disorder in Adults: Practical Help for Sufferers and Their Spouses*. Dallas: Taylor, 1992.
One of the first books on the topic, it contains a number of useful tips, questions, and answers. There is also a companion workbook with many exercises for the ADD adult.

Wender, Paul, M.D. *Attention Deficit Hyperactivity Disorder in Adults*. New York: Oxford University Press, 1995.
This book, designed for the professional, is technical

and academic. It contains what is probably the most thorough review of research on the etiology of ADD. Note that Wender's view that hyperactivity must be present for a diagnosis of ADD in adults is not universally accepted.

Wender, Paul, M.D. *The Hyperactive Child, Adolescent, and Adult*. New York: Oxford University Press, 1987.
   A good overview of ADD through the life span. Some sections are technical.

Videos

ADHD in Adults, by Russell Barkley. New York: Guilford Press, 1994.

Adults with Attention Deficit, by T. Phelan. Glen Ellyn, Ill: Child Management, Inc., 1994.

ADD Materials

Local Bookstores
(The manager will usually order for you a book that is not in stock.)

A.D.D. Plus
1095-25th Street SE #107
Salem, OR 97301
503-364-9163

ADD Warehouse
300 NW 70th Avenue, Suite 102
Plantation, FL 33317
800-233-9273
305-792-8960

Software and Videotapes

Center for Attention & Hyperactivity Disorders
2129 Belcourt Avenue
Nashville, TN 37212
615-383-1222

References

The following references cite primarily books and articles in scientific and academic journals aimed at professionals in the field of ADD. They also include some books and articles of interest to the general reader.

"Adults with ADHD May Pass Disorder to Their Children." *The Brown University Child and Adolescent Behavior Letter*. 11, no. 4 (April 1995): 6–7.

Alexander-Roberts, Colleen. *ADHD and Teens: A Parent's Guide to Making It Through the Tough Years*. Dallas: Taylor Publishing Company, 1995.

American Psychiatric Association. *Diagnostic and Statistical Manual of Mental Disorders, 4th Edition*. Washington, D.C.: Author, 1994.

Anderson, Peter D. "ADD Medicines and Driving." *The Med-ADD Review* 1, no. 3: 1–3.

———. "Controls on ADHD Drug Should Be Reduced" (editorial). *American Pharmacy*, NS34, no. 9 (September 1994): 5.

"Attention Deficit Disorder—Part I." *The Harvard Mental Health Letter* 11 (May 1995): 1–4.

"Attention Deficit Hyperactivity Disorder: Not Just for Kids." *Mayo Clinic Health Letter* 13 (September 1995): 6–7.

Barkley, Russell A. *Attention Deficit Hyperactivity Disorder: A Handbook for Diagnosis and Treatment*. New York: Guilford Press, 1990.

――――. "Is EEG Biofeedback Treatment Effective for ADD Children? Proceed with Much Caution." *Chadder Box*, April 1992, pp. 5–11.

――――. *Taking Charge of ADHD: The Complete Authoritative Guide for Parents*. New York: Guilford Press, 1995.

Barkley, R. A.; Guevremont, D. C.; Anastopoulos, A. D.; DuPaul, G. J.; and Shelton, T. L. "Driving-Related Risks and Outcomes of Attention Deficit Hyperactivity Disorder in Adolescents and Young Adults: A 3- to 5-Year Follow-Up Survey." *Pediatrics* 92 (1993): 212–18.

Berry, C. A.; Shaywitz, S. E.; and Shaywitz, B. A. "Girls with Attention Deficit Disorder: A Silent Minority? A Report on Behavioral and Cognitive Characteristics." *Pediatrics* 76, no. 5 (1985): 801–810.

Biederman, Joseph. "Current Research on Adult ADD." Cassette recording. CH.A.D.D. Conference, 1995

――――. "Gender Issues in ADD Adults." Paper presented at the Attention Deficit Information Network Conference, Waltham, Mass., May 1995. (For tape, call 603-534-6725.)

Biederman, Joseph; Faraone, Stephen V.; Mick, Eric; Spencer, Thomas; Wilens, Timothy; Kiely, Kathleen; Guite, Jessica; Ablon, J. Stuart; Reed, Ellen; and Warburton, Rebecca. "High Risk for Attention Deficit Hyperactivity Disorder Among Children of Parents with Childhood Onset of This Disorder: A Pilot Study." *American Journal of Psychiatry* 152 (March 1995): 431–36.

Biederman, Joseph; Faraone, Stephen V.; Spencer, Thomas; Wilens, Timothy; Norman, Denis; Lapey, Kathleen; Mick, Eric; Lehman, Belinda K.; and Doyle, Alysa. "Patterns of Psychiatric Comorbidity, Cognition, and Psychosocial Functioning in Adults with Attention Deficit Disorder," *American Journal of Psychiatry* 150 (December 1993): 1792–99.

Biederman, Joseph; Silver, Larry; Spencer, Thomas; Swanson,

Jon; and Wilens, Tim. "Current Issues of Pharmacological Treatment of ADD and Related Conditions in Children, Adolescents and Adults." Cassette recording. CH.A.D.D. Conference, 1995.

Biederman, Joseph; Faraone, Stephen V.; Spencer, Thomas; Wilens, Timothy; and Lapey, Kathleen. "Gender Differences in a Sample of Adults with Attention Deficit Hyperactivity Disorder." *Psychiatry Research* 53 (July 1994): 13–29.

Bower, Bruce. "Hyperactivity Grows into Adult Problems." *Science News* 144, no. 5 (July 31, 1993): 70–71.

Brown, David. "Childhood Hyperactivity Disorder Linked to Gene. *The Washington Post*, April 8, 1993, pp. A1–A2.

Brown, Thomas. "Complicated ADDs Without Hyperactivity: A Wide Umbrella Concept." Cassette recording. CH.A.D.D. Conference, 1995.

Brown, Thomas. "Differential Diagnosis of ADD Versus ADHD in Adults." In Nadeau, Kathleen G. *A Comprehensive Guide to Attention Deficit Disorder in Adults* (1994), pp. 93–108.

Castellanos, F. Xavier; Giedd, Jay N.; Eckburg, Paul; Marsh, Wendy L.; Vaituzis, Catherine, A.; Kaysen, Debra; Hamburger, Susan D.; and Rapoport, Judith L. "Quantitative Morphology of the Caudate Nucleus in Attention Deficit Hyperactivity Disorder." *American Journal of Psychiatry* 151 (1994): 1791–97.

"Cause of Attention-Deficit Hyperactivity Disorder." *American Family Physician* 49, no. 2 (February 1994): 460–62.

CH.A.D.D. Children and Adults with Attention Deficit Disorder. Proceedings of the CH.A.D.D. 1994 Annual Conference: Attention Deficit Disorders: A Global Perspective, New York City, October 13–15, 1994.

CH.A.D.D. "Controversial Treatments for Children with ADD." *CH.A.D.D. Facts*, no. 6 (1993).

Cohen, L.A.M. "Americans with Disabilities Act and Its Impact for People with ADD." *Challenge*, Winter 1995 (reprint).

Comings, E. "Adult Attention Deficit Disorder: Underdiagnosed, Undertreated." Nutrition Health Review, no. 63 (Summer 1992): 4–7.

Denckla, Martha B. "Attention Deficit Disorder—Residual Type." Journal of Child Neurology 6, Supplement (1991).

_____. "Learning and Producing Problems of Individuals with ADHD." Cassette recording. CH.A.D.D. Conference, 1995.

Ditter, Bob. "ADD/ADHD and Tourette Syndrome." Camping Magazine 67 (January–February 1995): 17–19.

Faraone, Stephen V.; Biederman, Joseph; Keenan, Kate; and Tsuang, Ming T. "A Family-Genetic Study of Girls with DSM-III Attention Deficit Disorder." American Journal of Psychiatry 148 (January 1991): 112–18.

Fargason, Rachel Epstein; and Ford, Charles F. "Attention Deficit Hyperactivity Disorder in Adults: Diagnosis, Treatment, and Prognosis." Southern Medical Journal 87 (March 1994): 302–309.

Farley, Dixie. "Helping Children with Attention Disorder." FDA Consumer 23 (February 1989): 10–15.

Feingold, Benjamin. Why Is Your Child Hyperactive? New York: Random House, 1975.

Gower, Timothy. "Attention Headache." Men's Health 9 (September 1994): 54–56.

Hales, Dianne; and Hales, Robert E. Caring for the Mind: The Comprehensive Guide to Mental Health. New York: Bantam Books, 1995.

_____. "Pay Attention: Hyperactivity Isn't Just for Children Anymore." American Health 12 (September 1993): 62–64.

Hallowell, Edward M.; and Ratey, John J. Driven to Distraction. New York: Pantheon, 1994.

Hartmann, Thom. Attention Deficit Disorder: A Different Perception. Novato, Calif: Underwood-Miller, 1993.

"Hyperactivity Disorder in Adults." Patient Care, February 28, 1989, pp. 21–23.

Jaffe, P. "I Was a Neurofeedback Trainee." *ADDendum* 9 (Summer 1992): 1–5.

Jensen, Peter S.; Shervette, Robert E., III; Xenais, Stephen; and Richters, John. "Anxiety and Depressive Disorders in Attention Deficit Disorder with Hyperactivity: New Findings." *American Journal of Psychiatry* 150 (August 1993): 1203–1210.

Kane, Robert; Mikalac, Cecilia; Benjamin, Sheldon; and Barkley, Russell, A. "Assessment and Treatment of Adults with ADHD." In *Attention Deficit Hyperactivity Disorder: A Handbook for Diagnosis and Treatment*, ed. Russell Berkley. New York: The Guilford Press, 1990.

Kelly, Kate. "Discovering Your ADD After All These Years: The Grief Process and Recovery." Cassette recording (tape no. 9). "The Changing World of Adults with ADD." Adult ADD Conference, Ann Arbor, 1993.

Kelly, Kate; and Ramundo, Peggy. *You Mean I'm Not Lazy, Stupid or Crazy?! A Self-Help Book for Adults with Attention Deficit Disorder*. Cincinnati: Tyrell and Jerem Press, 1993.

Kirkpatrick, Robert G., III. "Coaching the ADD Brain—A Perfect Prescription: An Interview with John Ratey, M.D." *Coaching Matters* 1 (Winter 1995): 2–4

Lahey, B. and Carlson, C. "Validity of the Diagnostic Category of Attention Deficit Disorder Without Hyperactivity." *Journal of Learning Disabilities*, 24(3), 110–20, 1991.

Lahey, B. B.; et al. "DSM-IV Trials for Attention Deficit Hyperactivity Disorder in Children and Adolescents." *American Journal of Psychiatry* 151 (1994): 1673–85.

Latham, Patricia H.; and Latham, Peter. "ADD in the Workplace." *Proceedings of the CH.A.D.D. 1994 Annual Conference*, Plantation, Fl., 1995.

Latham, Peter S.; and Latham, Patricia H. *Attention Deficit Disorder and the Law*. Washington, D.C.: JKL Communications, 1992.

McDonald, James J. Jr.; Kulick, Francine B.; and Creighton, Myra K. "Mental Disabilities Under the ADA: A Management Rights Approach." *Employee Relations Law Journal* 20 (Spring 1995): 541–70.

Mannuzza, Salvator; Klein, Rachel G.; Bessier, Abrah; Malloy, Patricia; and LaPadula, Maria. "Adult Outcome of Hyperactive Boys: Educational Achievement, Occupational Rank, and Psychiatric Status." *Archives of General Psychiatry* 50 (July 1993): 565–77.

Marshall-Cohen, Lei Ann. "Americans with Disabilities Act and Its Impact for People with ADD." *Attention!* (Winter 1995) (reprint, unpaginated).

Matochik, John A.; Liebenauer, M. A.; King, Catherine; Szymanksi, Herman V.; Cohen, Robert M.; and Zametkin, Alan J. "Cerebral Glucose Metabolism in Adults with Attention Deficit Hyperactivity Disorder after Chronic Stimulant Treatment." *American Journal of Psychiatry* 151, no. 5 (1994): 658–65.

Mattes, J. A. "Comparative Effectiveness of Carbamazapine and Propranolol for Rage Outbursts." *Journal of Neuropsychiatry and Clinical Neurosciences* 2, no. 2 (1990): 159–64.

Morgan, Babette. "How to Organize Your Mind: Pro Organizers Reveal Secrets of Being Neat." *St. Louis Post-Dispatch*, January 2, 1995.

Munoz, Millan; Robinson, J.; and Casteel, C. Richard. "Attention-Deficit Hyperactivity Disorder: Recent Literature." *Hospital and Community Psychiatry* 40 (July 1989): 699–705.

Murphy, Kevin R.; and LeVert, Suzanne. *Out of the Fog: Treatment Options and Coping Strategies for Adult Attention Deficit Disorder*. New York: Skylight Press, 1995.

Nadeau, Kathleen G. *A Comprehensive Guide to Attention Deficit Disorder in Adults.* New York: Brunner/Mazel, 1995.

———. *Survival Guide for College Students with ADD or LD*. New York: Magination Press, 1994.

National Institute of Mental Health. "Attention Deficit Hyperactivity Disorder" (pamphlet), September 1994, pp. 1–43.

"Q&A: An Interview with Judith Rapoport, M.D." *Attention!* 2, no. 3 (1996): 7–10.

Quinn, Patricia. "Psychopharmacological Treatment of Adolescents and Young Adults with ADD." Cassette Recording. CH.A.D.D. Conference, Washington, D.C., 1995.

Ratey, John J.; Miller, Andrea C.; and Nadeau, Kathleen G. "Special Diagnostic and Treatment Considerations in Women with Attention Deficit Disorder." In *A Comprehensive Guide to Attention Deficit Disorder in Adults*, ed. Kathleen G. Nadeau. New York: Brunner/Mazel, 1995.

Reisinger, Jim. "Blinks: An Unknown Attention Deficit Disorder." *ADDendum* 3 (Winter 1991): 4–5.

Royal, Weld F. "Sales and the Disease of the Information Age." *Sales & Marketing Management* 146 (August 1994): 59–61.

Shaffer, David. "Attention Deficit Hyperactivity Disorder in Adults" (editorial). *American Journal of Psychiatry* 151 (May 1994): 633–39.

Shaywitz, S. E.; and Shaywitz, B. D. "Attention Deficit Disorder: Current Perspectives." *Pediatric Neurology* 3 (May/June 1987): 129–35.

Shekim, Walid. "Residual Attention Deficit Disorder." *The Western Journal of Medicine* 151 (September 1989): 314–15.

Shekim, Walid O.; Asarnow, Robert F.; Hess, Esther; Zaucha, Ken; and Wheeler, Noel. "A Clinical and Demographic Profile of a Sample of Adults with Attention Deficit Hyperactivity Disorder, Residual State." *Comprehensive Psychiatry* 31 (September–October 1990): 416–26.

Silver, L. *Dr. Larry Silver's Advice to Parents on Attention Deficit Disorder*. Washington, D.C.: Psychiatric Press, 1993.

Solden, Sari. *Women with Attention Deficit Disorder*. Grass Valley, Calif.: Underwood Books, 1995.

Spencer, Thomas; Wilens, Timothy; Biederman, Joseph; Faraone, Stephen V.; Ablon, J. Stuart; and Lapey, Kathleen. "A Double-Blind, Crossover Comparison of Methylphenidate and Placebo in Adults with Childhood-

Onset Attention Deficit Hyperactivity Disorder." *Archives of General Psychiatry* 52 (June 1995): 434–54.

Stich, Sally. "Why Can't Your Husband Sit Still?" *Ladies Home Journal*, September 1993, pp. 74–76.

Stuart, Peggy. "Tracing Workplace Problems to Hidden Disorders." *Personnel Journal* 71 (June 1992): 82–91.

"Synthetic Food Colorings: Do They Affect Children's Behavior?" *Child Health Alert* 13 (February 1995): 1–3.

Szpir, Michael. "Alcoholism, Personality and Dopamine." *American Scientist* 83 (September–October 1995): 425–27.

Taibbi, Robert. "Understanding ADHD: More Than Just Active." *Current Health* 21 (March 1995): 16–18.

Taylor, Deborah Seymour. "Handle Hyperactivity with Dietary Measures." *Better Nutrition* 51 (August 1989): 14–16.

United States Pharmacopeial Convention, Inc. *Advice for the Patient: Drug Information in Lay Language.* USP DI-Vol. II, Edition 15 (1995).

"Urinary Catecholamines in ADHD with Anxiety." *The Brown University Child and Adolescent Behavior Letter* 11, no. 8 (August 1995): 6–7.

Verbaten, M. N.; Overtoom, C.C.E.; Koelega, H. S.; Swaab-Barneveld, H.; Gaag, R. J. van der; Buitelaar J.; and Engeland, H. van. "Methylphenidate Influences on Both Early and Late ERP Waves of ADHD Children in a Continuous Performance Test." *Journal of Abnormal Child Psychology* 22 (October 1994): 561–69.

Wallace, Amy E.; Kofoed, Lial L.; and West, Alan N. "Double-Blind, Placebo-Controlled Trial of Methylphenidate in Older, Depressed, Medically Ill Patients." *American Journal of Psychiatry* 152 (June 1995): 929–32.

Wallis, Claudia. "Life in Overdrive." *Time,* July 18, 1994, pp. 42–51.

Ward, Mark, F.; Wender, Paul H.; and Reimherr, Fred W. "The Wender Utah Rating Scale: An Aid in the Retrospective Diagnosis of Childhood Attention Deficit Hyperactivity Disorder." *American Journal of Psychiatry* 150 (June 1993): 885–91.

Warren, Reed P.; Odell, J. Dennis; Warren, W. Louise; Burger, Roger A.; Maciulis, Alma; and Torres, Anthony R. "Is Decreased Blood Plasma Concentration of the Complement C4B Protein Associated with Attention-Deficit Hyperactivity Disorder." *Psychiatry* 34 (August 1995): 1009–1015:

Weiss, Gabrielle; and Hechtman, Lily Trokenberg. *Hyperactive Children Grown Up: ADHD in Children, Adolescents, and Adults.* New York: The Guilford Press, 1993.

Wender, Paul. *Attention Deficit Hyperactivity Disorder in Adults.* New York: Oxford University Press, 1995.

———. *The Hyperactive Child, Adolescent, and Adult: Attention Deficit Disorder Through the Lifespan.* New York: Oxford University Press, 1987.

Wender, Paul H.; and Reimherr, Fred W. "Bupruprion Treatment of Attention-Deficit Hyperactivity Disorder in Adults." *American Journal of Psychiatry* 147 (August 1990): 1018–21.

White, M. "What Adults with ADD Would Like Their Friends, Relatives and Others to Know." *Challenge* Vol. 8 no. 4: 109.

Whiteman, T. A.; and Novotny, M. *Adult ADD.* Colorado Springs: Pinion Press, 1995.

Wilens, Timothy. "Advanced Psychopharmacotherapy of ADD." Cassette recording. CH.A.D.D. Conference, Washington, D.C., 1995.

Wilens, Timothy; Biederman, Joseph; Spencer, Thomas J.; and Prince, Jefferson. "Pharmacotherapy of Adult Attention Deficit/Hyperactivity Disorder: A Review." *Journal of Clinical Psychopharmacology* 15 (August 1995): 270–79.

Wilens, Timothy; Biederman, Joseph; Spencer, Thomas J. "Pharmacotherapy of Adult ADHD." In Nadeau, Kathleen G. *A Comprehensive Guide to Attention Deficit Disorder in Adults* (1994), pp. 168–88.

Wilens, Timothy; Biederman, Joseph; Mick, Eric; and Spencer, Thomas. "A Systematic Assessment of Tricyclic Antidepressants in the Treatment of Adult Attention-Deficit

Hyperactivity Disorder." *Journal of Nervous and Mental Disease* 183 (1995): 48–51.

Wolraich, Mark L.; Wlson, David B.; and White, J. Wade. "The Effect of Sugar on Behavior or Cognition in Children: A Meta-Analysis." *JAMA: The Journal of the American Medical Association* 274 (November 22, 1995): 1617–22.

Zametkin, Alan J. "Attention-Deficit Disorder: Born to Be Hyperactive?" *JAMA: The Journal of the American Medical Association* 273 (June 21, 1995): 1871–75.

Zane, J. Peder. "Neatness Counts, and They're Out to Prove It: Professional Organizers Clean Up Your Act if You Can't Do it Yourself." *The New York Times*, May 7, 1995.

About the Authors

James Lawrence Thomas, Ph.D., is a psychologist and neuropsychologist with postdoctoral certificates in neuropsychology, cognitive therapy, relationship therapy, group and brief therapy. He is on the faculty of New York University Medical Center and has served as consulting neuropsychologist to the Department of Neurology at Mount Sinai Medical Center in New York City.

During the last twenty years Dr. Thomas has treated many children and adults with ADD, using a variety of the methods and treatments described in this book. He is fascinated by ADD and continues to learn from his patients. He is also ADD himself and thus understands the disorder from the inside.

"I like to work in a collaborative way to empower the adult with ADD and to discover the real person inside," he says. "I want to help the person develop his or her strengths, and even shine, as he or she learns how to cope with this troublesome condition that we call attention deficit disorder."

Christine A. Adamec is a freelance writer from Palm Bay, Florida. She has written five books, including three published in 1996: *There ARE Babies to Adopt; When Your Pet Dies;* and *How to Live with a Mentally Ill Person*. Her earlier books are *The Encyclopedia of Adoption* (1991) and *Start and Run a Profitable Freelance Writing Business* (1994). She has also written hundreds of feature articles.

Ms. Adamec has a bachelor's degree in psychology and an MBA in business management.

Index